CARDIOPULMONARY
PHYSIOTHERAPY

CARDIOPULMONARY PHYSIOTHERAPY

M Jones (Ph.D., MCSP)
Royal Brompton and Harefield NHS Trust, UK

and

F Moffatt (M.Sc., MCSP)
Queen's Medical Centre Nottingham
(University Hospital NHS Trust), UK

A CIP catalogue record for this book is available from the British Library.

ISBN 1 85996 297 1

BIOS Scientific Publishers Ltd
9 Newtec Place, Magdalen Road, Oxford OX4 1RE, UK
Tel. +44 (0)1865 726286. Fax +44 (0)1865 246823
World Wide Web home page: http://www.bios.co.uk/

IMPORTANT NOTE FROM THE PUBLISHER
The information contained within this book was obtained by BIOS Scientific Publishers Ltd from sources believed by us to be reliable. However, while every effort has been made to ensure its accuracy, no responsibility for loss or injury whatsoever occasioned to any person acting or refraining from action as a result of information contained herein can be accepted by the authors or publishers.

The reader should remember that medicine is a constantly evolving science and while the authors and publishers have ensured that all dosages, applications and practices are based on current indications, there may be specific practices which differ between communities. You should always follow the guidelines laid down by the manufacturers of specific products and the relevant authorities in the country in which you are practising.

Production Editor: Andrew Watts
Typeset by Phoenix Photosetting, Chatham, Kent
Printed by Biddles Ltd, Guildford, UK

CONTENTS LIST

ACKNOWLEDGMENTS

The authors wish to acknowledge the valuable contributions made by Dr Andy Jones to the pathophysiology section and Andrew Love to the pain chapter. Grateful thanks to Frank Makin and Rupert Murch for their technical support.

Thanks, as always to our families for providing the time, encouragement and babysitting which has enabled us to write this text.

MJ & FM

ABBREVIATIONS

ABG	arterial blood gas
ACBT	active cycle of breathing techniques
ACE-inhibitor	angiotensin-converting enzyme inhibitor
AD	autogenic drainage
ADH	anti-diuretic hormone
AIDS	acquired immune deficiency syndrome
ALI	acute lung injury
AP	anteroposterior
ARDS	acute respiratory distress syndrome
BE	base excess
BiPAP	bi-phasic (or bi-level) positive airway pressure
BP	blood pressure
bpm	beats per minute
BS	breath sound
C4	4th cervical vertebra
°C	degrees centigrade
CAL	chronic airflow limitation
CAPD	continuous ambulatory peritoneal dialysis
CC	closing capacity
CCF	congestive cardiac failure
CHF	congestive heart failure
CF	cystic fibrosis
cmH_2O	centimeters of water
CMV	controlled mandatory ventilation
CO_2	carbon dioxide
CPAP	continuous positive airways pressure
CSF	cerebrospinal fluid
CSR	Cheyne–Stokes respiration
CT	computerized tomography
CVP	central venous pressure
CXR	chest x-ray
DH	drug history
DIC	disseminated intravascular coagulation
$ECCO_2R$	extra corporeal carbon dioxide removal
ECG	electrocardiogram
ECMO	extra corporeal membrane oxygenation
EEG	electro-encephalogram
EPAP	expiratory positive airway pressure
ETT	endotracheal tube
FET	forced expiration technique
FEV_1	forced expiratory volume in 1 second
FH	family history
F_iO_2	fraction of inspired oxygen

FRC	functional residual capacity
FVC	forced vital capacity
GA	general anesthesia
GAP	gravity-assisted positioning
GI	gastro-intestinal
GPB	glossopharyngeal breathing
GTN	glycerin trinitrate
H^+	hydrogen ions
Hb	hemoglobin
HCO_3^-	bicarbonate ions
HIV	human immunodeficiency virus
HME	heat & moisture exchanger
HPC	history of present condition
HPV	hypoxic pulmonary vasoconstriction
HR	heart rate
Hz	hertz
ICP	intracranial pressure
ICU	intensive care unit
IPAP	inspiratory positive airway pressure
IS	incentive spirometry
IPPB	intermittent positive pressure breathing
JVP	jugular venous pressure
K^+	potassium
Kcal	kilocalorie
KPa	kilopascals
L	left
L/day	litres per day
LIP	lower inflection point
LL	lower lobe
L/min	liters per minute
LTEE	lower thoracic expansion exercises
LTOT	long-term oxygen therapy
LVF	left ventricular failure
MAC	minimum alveolar concentration
MDI	metered dose inhaler
METs	metabolic equivalents
MHI	manual hyperinflation
MI	myocardial infarction
ML	middle lobe
ml/kg/hour	milliliters per kilogram per hour
mmHg	millimeters of mercury
mmol	millimols
MOF	multiple organ failure
MRI	magnetic resonance imaging
MRSA	methicillin-resistant *Staphylococcus aureus*
MV	mechanical ventilation

Na^+	sodium
NPF	neurophysiological facilitation of respiration
NIPPV	non-invasive positive pressure ventilation
NM	neuromuscular
NSAID	non-steroidal anti-inflammatory drugs
O_2	oxygen
O/E	on examination
PA	posteroanterior
P_aCO_2	partial pressure arterial carbon dioxide
P_ACO_2	partial pressure alveolar carbon dioxide
P_aO_2	partial pressure arterial oxygen
P_AO_2	partial pressure alveolar oxygen
PAOD	peripheral arterial obstructive disease
PAP	pulmonary artery pressure
PCAS	patient-controlled analgesia system
PCO_2	partial pressure carbon dioxide
PCOP	pulmonary capillary occlusion pressure
PE	pulmonary embolus
PEEP	positive end expiratory pressure
PEFR	peak expiratory flow rate
PEP	positive expiratory pressure
PH	previous history
P_iO_2	partial pressure of inspired oxygen
PO_2	partial pressure of oxygen
PSV	pressure support ventilation
PV	pressure–volume
RPE	rate of perceived exertion
R	right
RR	respiratory rate
SALT	speech & language therapist
S_aO_2	arterial oxygen saturation
Sec	seconds
SH	social history
SIMV	synchronized intermittent mandatory ventilation
SIRS	systemic inflammatory response syndrome
SNS	sympathetic nervous system
SOB	short of breath
SOBAR	short of breath at rest
SOBOE	short of breath on exertion
TB	tuberculosis
T_1	1st thoracic vertebra
TENS	transcutaneous electrical nerve stimulation
Trache	tracheostomy tube
UIP	upper inflection point
UL	upper lobe
VALI	ventilator-acquired lung injury

VC	vital capacity
VO_{2max}	maximal oxygen uptake
V_T	tidal volume
V/Q	ventilation/perfusion ratio
WBC	white blood cells
XR	x-ray

HOW TO USE THIS BOOK

With the advent of evidence-based clinical practice, there is no longer a place for routine cardiopulmonary physiotherapy. The 'recipe' approach to physiotherapy treatment is no longer acceptable. A treatment choice should be based upon several key steps; a thorough analytical assessment, the identification of specific pathophysiological problems followed by the application of clinical reasoning to select an appropriate physiotherapeutic intervention. It should be remembered that assessment is a continuing process, performed before, during and after any treatment.

An understanding of the physiological basis behind commonly encountered cardiopulmonary pathology is essential to enable the physiotherapist to make an informed choice in selecting suitable treatment modalities. This book has been designed to reflect today's clinical practice with sections on assessment, cardiopulmonary pathophysiology and physiotherapy techniques and adjuncts.

The aim of the text is to provide the physiotherapist with all the necessary assessment tools to assess any adult patient with cardiopulmonary dysfunction. The assessment procedure will identify clinical problems secondary to underlying or co-existent pathology. The pathophysiology section offers a succinct explanation of each pathophysiological process and gives the reader an understanding of its clinical relevance and implications. The physiotherapy techniques and adjuncts section presents a comprehensive range of physiotherapeutic interventions and skills, which can be used in the treatment of the identified problems. The physiological basis underlying the action of each treatment modality is explained, together with an evidence-based evaluation of its clinical efficacy. Using selected text from each section the physiotherapist may carry out an appropriate assessment, identify problems and apply clinical reasoning to devise an effective management plan. Topics are cross-referenced throughout the text to facilitate this process.

Case studies are provided at the end of the book as a self-assessment exercise.

This text is written as a quick reference pocket book, which may in part assume some pre-existing knowledge. Where necessary the reader is directed to other sources.

Section 1

ASSESSMENT TOOLS

ASSESSMENT TOOLS

Introduction

Respiratory examination must form part of a multisystem assessment, as physiologically no body system works in isolation. The clinician should review available medical/nursing documents and charts to insure that any overall 'trends' are identified, as this will prevent findings being taken out of context. Early detection of physiological changes may prevent catastrophic patient deterioration. Liaison with members of the multidisciplinary team will insure a holistic examination is performed.

This section provides all the core tools necessary for the physiotherapy assessment of any patient with a respiratory system disorder, from a simple pre-operative examination to the complex assessment of the critically ill patient. The physiotherapist must use their clinical judgment to select the appropriate assessment tools.

Assessment is an on-going procedure and should be performed before, during and after every treatment.

Subjective examination

- HPC including onset, progression, signs and symptoms, treatment/response, identification of problems as seen by the patient.

  DOES THE CURRENT CONDITION REPRESENT A CHANGE FROM NORMAL AND IF SO, HOW?

During assessment of the following signs and symptoms, identify the nature, precipitating factors, methods of relief, effect of treatment, diurnal variations, severity and associated symptoms:

- SOB: mild/moderate/severe (visual analog scale, Borg scale), orthopnea, and paroxysmal nocturnal dyspnea.
- Wheeze: PEFR ↑↓.
- Cough: productive, dry, nocturnal.
- Sputum: quantity, color, consistency, and hemoptysis.
- Exercise tolerance and functional limitations: descriptive terms (distance, pain, dyspnea, fatigue), stair climbing.
- Pain: body chart, visual analog scale, descriptive terms.
- Relevant PH, DH, SH, FH.

Objective examination

Central nervous system

	Intracranial pressure	Cerebral perfusion pressure
Normal value	<10 mmHg	>70 mmHg
Critical value	>25 mmHg	<50 mmHg

- Level of consciousness (Glasgow coma scale), orientation (time, person, place).
- Pupil size/reactivity/equality.
- Ability to maintain a patent airway.
- Sensorimotor loss, speech disturbances.
- Level of pain/agitation.
- Note results from interventions: transcerebral Doppler, CT scans, MRI scans, EEGs, cerebral function activity monitor.
- Note the presence and location of ventricular drains, bone flaps, jugular bulbs.
- Pharmacological support: muscle relaxants, sedatives, anxiolytic agents, anti-depressant agents, anesthetic agents, analgesics, osmotic diuretics, cerebral artery vasodilators, anticonvulsing agents and cortical steroids.

Cardiovascular system

	Heart rate (HR)	Arterial blood pressure (BP)	Central venous pressure (CVP)	Pulmonary artery pressure (PAP)	Pulmonary capillary occlusion pressure (PCOP)
Normal range	50–100 bpm	95–120/60–90 mmHg	3–15 mmHg	10–20 mmHg	6–15 mmHg
	bradycardia <50 bpm tachycardia >100 bpm		Note palpable JVP		

- Rhythm (normal sinus rhythm, abnormal, e.g. atrial fibrillation/flutter, ventricular tachycardia, ectopic beats, ventricular fibrillation, heart block).
- Note presence and severity of peripheral edema.
- Note presence and quality of peripheral pulses or signs of peripheral circulatory insufficiency.
- Note results of cardiac output studies: cardiac index, systemic/pulmonary vascular resistance, calculated values of right/left atrial pressure.
- Note presence of pulmonary artery catheter, central and arterial lines.
- Note presence and rate of drainage in mediastinal drains.
- Review relevant tests: 12-lead ECG, angiogram, echocardiogram, cardiac enzymes, exercise test (Bruce protocol).
- Pharmacological support: inotropes, antihypertensive agents, anti-arrhythmic agents, ACE inhibitors, vasodilators, diuretics, crystalloid, colloid, antithrombolytic and anticoagulant agents.
- Mode of mechanical support: ventricular assist devices, intra-aortic balloon pumps, pacemakers and inplantable defibrillators.

Respiratory system

- Mode of ventilation: spontaneous, assisted, intubated and ventilated, NIPPV.
- Level of PEEP, CPAP or pressure support.

- Respiratory rate: normal spontaneous 10–15 breaths per minute. In a ventilated patient respiratory rate may be widely manipulated to achieve different clinical objectives, e.g. hyperventilation with acute head injury. N.B. Respiratory rate change is commonly the most sensitive indicator of physiological deterioration.
- Respiratory pattern: work of breathing (at rest and with exercise), use of accessory muscles, pursed lip breathing, intercostal recession, paradoxical movement, Cheyne–Stokes respiration, apneustic breathing.
- Inspiration:expiration ratio (may be manipulated with mechanical ventilation to achieve different clinical objectives, e.g. prolonged inspiration to increase oxygenation, or prolonged expiration to minimize air trapping in obstructive lung disease).
- Airway pressures (peak and mean).
- Fraction of inspired oxygen (F_iO_2) and delivery device.
- Type of humidification device.
- Use of pulse oximetry or capnography.
- Presence and rate of drainage in intercostal drains.
- Shape of thorax: barrel, kyphosis, scoliosis, thoracoplasty and pectus cavinatum/excavatum.
- Color (e.g. cyanosis), nicotine stains and finger clubbing.
- Palpation: thoracic expansion, tracheal position and mobility, secretions, bony crepitus and surgical emphysema.
- Cough and sputum (nature of cough, color, viscosity, quantity and odor of sputum).
- Pharmacological support: oxygen, bronchodilator agents, mast-cell stabilizers, steroids, inflammatory cell antagonists, mucolytic agents, inhaled pulmonary vasodilators, inhaled antibiotics, respiratory stimulants and surfactant.
- Mechanical support: ECMO, $ECCO_2R$.

Auscultation
- Where possible always fully expose the thorax.
- Listen to a full inspiration and expiration (normal ratio 1:2).
- Note where in respiratory cycle any abnormality occurs, inspiration/expiration.
- Note where in inspiration/expiration abnormality occurs, early, middle or late.
- Listen over the trachea and main bronchi.
- Work down the lung fields comparing both sides:
  – upper lobe: apical, anterior and posterior segments;
  – middle/lingula lobes: medial and lateral/superior and inferior segments;
  – lower lobe: apical, medial, lateral, anterior and posterior segments.
- Breath sounds: normal, reduced or added.
- Normal: equal and bilateral.
- Reduced: consider atelectasis, collapse, pleural effusion, empyema, pneumothorax, hypoventilation, hyperinflation and absence of lung tissue.
- Added sounds:
  – Crackles: generated by opening of previously closed alveoli and small airways. Fine or coarse: fine, consider fibrosis or pulmonary edema, coarse, consider sputum.

– Wheeze: musical note generated by air vibrating a narrowed airway. Initially heard in expiration, can progress to inspiration. Monophonic or polyphonic; monophonic denotes single airway obstruction, consider sputum plug; polyphonic, denotes widespread airway involvement, consider bronchospasm.

– Pleural rub: creaking noise generated with articulation of inflamed pleura.

– Bronchial breath sounds: normal breath sounds heard over the trachea and main bronchi. However, can be transmitted and heard over airless areas of lung. Loud noise with harsh quality. Heard equally through inspiration and expiration with a short pause between the two phases. Consider consolidation, or a large area of obstruction.

– Stridor: upper airway or laryngeal obstruction. Potentially life-threatening situation. Physiotherapy contraindicated. Discuss with doctor immediately.

– Transmitted noise and artefact: note sounds occurring due to movement of stethoscope bell against bed sheets or skin. Mechanical sounds may be transmitted from a ventilator, nebulizer, intercostal drains or humidification device.

- Percussion note: generated by percussing the chest with one finger, to produce vibration of underlying chest wall and tissues. Always compare to normal aerated lung. Areas of reduced resonance sound dull, consider consolidation, pleural effusion, empyema or collapse/atelectasis. Areas which sound hyper-resonant, consider pneumothorax, emphysema.

- Vocal resonance: normal lung attenuates high frequency sound, transmitting low frequency only. Auscultate the chest wall whilst the patient repeats '99'. Increased resonance ('bleating' quality): consider consolidation, fibrosis, etc. This test may be repeated with the patient whispering '99' (whispering petriloquy), as whispered speech would not normally be detected by auscultation except over solid lung. N.B. Tactile vocal fremitus works on the same principle as vocal resonance, except the chest wall is palpated rather than auscultated.

Chest x-ray interpretation

- CXR adds an important dimension to clinical assessment, together with a review of patient history and examination findings.
- The technical quality of the CXR should be reviewed prior to clinical evaluation.
- CXR is anatomical thus cannot represent physiological changes, e.g. bronchospasm.
- CXR is a 2-D representation of a 3-D object.
- CXR may lag behind other clinical changes.

Physical background:

- CXR has the ability to penetrate matter, and this is dependent upon density.
- Dense structures absorb more rays, and less dense structures absorb less. Therefore adjacent structures of different densities have an identifiable border.
- The closer the structure to the source of the XR, the greater the magnification and distortion.

Indications:

- Detect alterations secondary to pathology.
- Trend the progression of lung disease.
- Determine therapy.

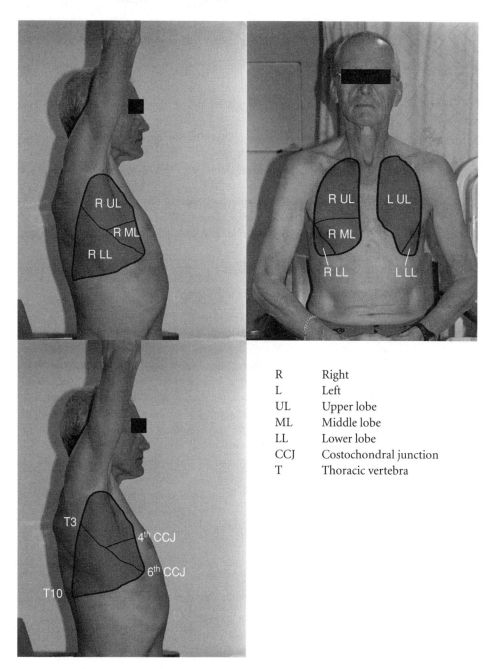

R   Right
L   Left
UL   Upper lobe
ML   Middle lobe
LL   Lower lobe
CCJ   Costochondral junction
T   Thoracic vertebra

Figure 1. Surface markings of the lungs (approximate).

- Evaluate effectiveness of treatment.
- Determine position of tubes and catheters.

Terminology:

- Silhouette sign: An obliteration of the border of the heart/mediastinum/hemidiaphragm by an adjacent opacity. Allows the clinician to localize lesions, e.g. a lesion in the right lung obscuring part of the heart border must be in the right middle lobe. If the lesion obscures the border of the hemidiaphragm, it is in the right lower lobe.
- Zones: A useful tool for describing location of lesions, although it does not give information regarding lobes.
  – Upper zone: above the right anterior border of the 2nd rib.
  – Mid zone: between right anterior borders of 2nd and 4th ribs.
  – Lower zone: between right anterior border of 4th rib and the hemidiaphragm.

Table 1. Technical evaluation of a CXR.

Technical evaluation	Assessment	Consequence
Rotation	Spinous processes central Clavicles symmetrical	Structures will appear shifted
Penetration	Vertebral bodies just visible through heart shadow	Overexposed = black lungs, underexposed = white lungs
Depth of inspiration	Midpoint of R hemidiaphragm should be between 5th and 7th ribs anteriorly	Broader mediastinum, elevated hemidiaphragm if inadequate inspiration
Entire chest on film	Laterally and vertically	Essential for accurate diagnosis
Film on viewer correctly	Check L & R	Essential for accurate diagnosis
Correct patient/date	Check label	Essential for accurate diagnosis and evaluating series of XR
Erect or supine	Check labeling	Hemidiaphragm higher, mediastinum wider on supine
Projection	Scapular shadow seen on AP Heart shadow larger on an AP	May need to modify interpretation

Clinical evaluation:

- Airway (trachea, carina, deviation, strictures, ETT, etc.);
- bones and soft tissues (ribs, scapulae, vertebrae, density, fractures, etc.);

- cardiac shadow, mediastinum and hilum (cardiac size/borders/orientation, major vessels, hilar enlargement/deviation/shape etc.);
- diaphragm and lung fields (hemidiaphragm height/borders, costophrenic and cardiophrenic angles, fissure, lung markings, transradiency, etc.).

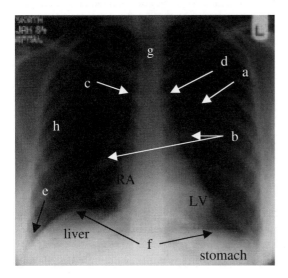

a lung markings
b hilar shadows
c mediastinum
d aortic knuckle
e costophrenic angle
f hemidiaphragm
g trachea
h approx position horiz. fissure
RA right atrium
LV left ventricle

Figure 2. Anatomical landmarks of a normal CXR.

Common radiological problems

Atelectasis or collapse

- Signifies loss of air in a portion of lung.
- Direct displacement of fissures, pulmonary blood vessels, major bronchi and trachea. Shift of other structures to compensate, e.g. overexpansion of adjacent lobe, mediastinal shift (greatest in LL collapse, mild with UL and minimal with ML) or elevated hemidiaphragm (especially right/left LL collapse or left UL).
- Right UL collapse: the fissure moves up and the right UL impacts against mediastinum and lung apex.
- Left UL collapse: a hazy density extending from the left hilum towards the apex, fading inferiorly and laterally. The silhouette sign (i.e. extent of cardiac and upper mediastinal border) depends upon the extent of left LL overexpansion.
- Right ML collapse: loss of the silhouette of the right heart border. It is easily recognized on a lateral, where the horizontal and oblique fissures approximate.
- Right LL collapse: a triangular opacity based on the diaphragm and mediastinum, with the fissure running obliquely through the thorax.
- Left LL collapse: the 'flat waist' represents a flattening of the contours of the aortic knuckle and adjacent pulmonary artery. The heart shadow will appear much whiter then normal, and a white triangle may be seen behind it.
- Whole lung collapse: opacity of the whole hemithorax and compensatory shift.
- Plate or discoid atelectasis: result of peripheral pulmonary collapse. It is due to hypoventilation and is especially common in postoperative patients.

Airspace shadowing (consolidation)
- Radiographic appearance that implies replacement of air in distal airways and alveoli, by fluid or other material, e.g. pneumonia, infarction, contusion, aspiration.
- Shadowing in lung fields (not uniform) with poorly demarcated border (except where abutting the pleura or mediastinum). Presence of air bronchogram (area of radiolucency within airspace shadowing).

Pneumothorax
- Loss of negative pressure in the pleural space, therefore the lungs' normal elasticity is unopposed.
- Unilateral black lung (not related to technical problem or mastectomy) with visible lung edge.
- Loss of lung markings (i.e. absence of vascular shadows).
- Surgical emphysema may be present.
- Will be more pronounced in an expiratory film.

Hyperinflation
- Lungs inflated above and beyond normal physiological volumes.
- Large lung volume (able to count more than seven ribs anteriorly) with flattened hemidiaphragm and spindle heart.
- Enlarged intercostal spaces and increased transradiancy due to reduced lung markings.

CCF
- Cardiac failure associated with pulmonary edema.
- UL diversion (enlarged, prominent blood vessels in UL where they should be small and barely noticeable). Applies only to an erect film; UL diversion is normal in supine films.
- Increased heart size (may not occur in acute-onset LVF).
- Kerley B lines if PCOP >25 mmHg (horizontal, non-branching lines seen peripherally at the base, caused by edema of interlobular septa).
- Increased interstitial markings and hilar engorgement ('bat's wing shadowing').

Pleural effusion
- Collection of transudate or exudate in pleural space. A total of 100 cc must collect before it can be seen on CXR.
- Blunting of costophrenic angle with visible meniscal edge often seen in an erect film.
- Partially obscured hemidiaphragmy, to white out with completely obscured hemidiaphragm.
- May be loculated.

Coin lesions
- An area of opacity located within the lung field, e.g. tumor, infection, infarction.
- Irregular edge is suggestive of malignancy.
- Look for other associated abnormalities, e.g. distal collapse, effusions or consolidation.

Ring shadows and cysts

- Caused by many factors, e.g. abscess, neoplasms, airway disease.
- Bullae: black densities surrounded by fine ring shadow.
- 'String of pearls' or 'bunch of grapes' in bronchiectasis.
- May contain an air/fluid level.
- May be 'mimicked' by bowel herniation or plombage.

Widespread reticular shadowing

- Nodular; clearly defined opacities, e.g. miliary TB, sarcoidosis.
- Cystic; widespread ring shadows, e.g. CF.
- Reticular; fine linear shadowing, e.g. pulmonary edema.
- Reticular-nodular; mesh of lines converging to form ring shadows and nodules, e.g. fibrosis.

ABG analysis

- Normal values:

pH	7.35–7.45	
$[H^+]$	36–44 nmol/l	
PO_2	10.5–14 kPa (70–100 mmHg)	
PCO_2	4.5–6 kPa (35–46 mmHg)	
HCO_3^-	22–26 mmol/l	
BE	−2 – +2	
SaO_2	>95%	

- The normal range for pH is 7.35–7.45, however, neutral is 7.4. Therefore any value above 7.4 is alkaline and any below 7.4 is acid even if within the normal range.
- The concentration of H^+ ions is a more accurate indication of acidity/alkalinity.
- The value of PO_2 has no influence on acidity/alkalinity.
- PCO_2 can change rapidly whereas HCO_3^- may take several days to alter.
- PCO_2 is an acid, therefore values above normal range indicate a respiratory acidosis and values below normal range indicate a respiratory alkalosis.
- The normal range for HCO_3^- is 22–26 mmol/l, however, neutral is 25 mmol/l.
- HCO_3^- is an alkali, therefore values above 25 mmol/l indicate a metabolic alkalosis and below 25 mmol/l indicate a metabolic acidosis.
- The body aims to keep respiratory acidity and metabolic alkalinity in constant balance. Therefore, a primary alteration in one often leads to a secondary compensatory change in the other.
- The system (respiratory/PCO_2 or metabolic/HCO_3^-) which shows a derangement in the same direction as the pH (acid or alkali) is the primary cause of the problem. A compensatory change should occur in the other system to maintain acid–base balance. Full compensation is said to have occurred when pH values within normal range are achieved.

After reviewing all clinical data:

- Firstly look at the pH – ? acidosis/alkalosis (7.4).
- Next look at PCO_2 – ? increased/decreased/normal (4.5–6).
- Do the pH and the PCO_2 show the same thing (acidity/alkalinity)?
- Is there a primary respiratory problem or is this the compensatory change?

- Is the compensation full or partial?
- Now look at the HCO_3^- – ? increased/decreased/normal (25)
- Do the pH and the HCO_3^- show the same thing (acidity/alkalinity)?
- Is this the primary problem or the compensatory change?
- Is the compensation full or partial?

Spirometry

Indications

- To define an abnormality.
- To monitor disease progression.
- To indicate response to a treatment.
- Pre-operative assessment.

Considerations
- Age.
- Sex.
- Stature/posture.
- Fitness.
- Diurnal variations.

Peak expiratory flow rate (PEFR)

- Easily repeatable and portable test which reflects variability in airway caliber.
- Normal range 300–600 l/min.

More accurate and reproducible than PEFR

- (F)VC – the total volume of gas that can be exhaled after full inspiration.
- Prefix F, indicates a forced expiratory maneuver.
- FEV_1 – volume of gas exhaled in 1 second after a full inspiration, during a forced expiratory maneuver.
- FEV_1/FVC – the proportion of the FVC exhaled in the 1st second.
- Normal: 75–80%.
- Obstructive lung disease (asthma, CAL): <75%
  – Implies impaired lung emptying:
     <75% = mild;
     <60% = moderate;
     <40% = severe.
- Restrictive lung disease (pulmonary fibrosis, NM disorders): >80%
  – Implies impaired expansion with preserved emptying.

Peak flow and spirometry recordings represent simple measures of lung function that can be easily and repeatedly performed at the bedside. For a more accurate assessment of pulmonary function, a more elaborate series of tests exist, normally performed in the lung function laboratory.

Immune system, hematology and microbiology

	Core body temperature	Full blood count	Clotting profile
Normal value	36–37.5°C	Hemoglobin 12–17 g/dl	Activated clotting time 100–140 s
		Mean corpuscular volume 76–96 fl	Thrombin time 12–16 s
		White cell count 4–11 × 10⁹/l	Prothrombin time 12–16 s
		Platelets 150–400 × 10⁹/l	Activated partial thromboblastin time 30–40 s
			d-dimers and fibrin degradation products <10 μg/ml

- External signs of infection, e.g. infected wounds, foul-smelling sputum.
- Review microbiology, serology and virology results; e.g. blood cultures, sputum specimens, bronchoalveolar lavage, mid-stream urine, MRSA status, HIV status, etc.
- Pharmacological support, e.g.: antibiotics, antiviral and antifungal agents, paracetamol, anticoagulants, blood products, crystalloid and colloid, cytotoxic agents, immunosuppressant drugs, etc.

Renal system

	Urine output	Electrolytes	Acid–base balance
Normal value	0.5 ml/kg/hour Anuria – no urine output Oliguria <0.5 ml/kg/hour Polyuria >2 l/day	Urea 3–8 mmol/l Creatinine 50–120 μmol/l Sodium 134–146 mmol/l Potassium 3.4–5 mmol/l Calcium 2.2–2.6 mmol/l	pH 7.35–7.45 Bicarbonate 22–26 mmol/l Base excess ±2

- Fluid balance (possible peripheral/pulmonary edema or ascites with a large positive fluid balance, impaired mucociliary clearance and hemodynamic insufficiency with a large negative balance).
- Impaired drug clearance occurs with renal failure.
- Presence and location of lines and cannulae for dialysis/hemofiltration.
- Pharmacological support, e.g. diuretic or inotropic agents.
- Mechanical support e.g.: hemodialysis, hemofiltration, continuous ambulatory peritoneal dialysis (CAPD), peritoneal dialysis.

GI tract and hepatic system

	Glucose	Liver function tests
Normal values	4–6 mmol/l	Albumin 35–53 g/l Bilirubin 3–17 µmol/l

- Evidence of GI dysfunction likely to affect cardiorespiratory system (e.g. abdominal sepsis, abdominal distention, vomiting, large nasogastric aspirates, etc.).
- Nutritional status including oral/enteral/parenteral diet.
- Abdominal scars/incisions/stoma.
- Presence of abdominal or rectal drains, nasogastric tubes, feeding lines, etc.
- Color (jaundice).
- Pharmacological support, e.g. gastric protection, anti-emetic agents, laxatives, antidiarrhea agents, and vitamin K.

Musculoskeletal system

- Mobility and muscle strength (joint movement, bed mobility, transfers, gait, stair climbing).
- Exercise tolerance (e.g. shuttle walk test, stair climbing).
- Bony or soft tissue injury/pathology.
- Use of walking aids, external fixation, specialized beds/equipment.
- Crepitus, e.g. rib fractures.
- Thoracic joint /glenohumeral joint mobility.
- Pharmacological support: NSAIDs, steroids, antispasmodic agents, bisphosphinates.

Risk assessment

- Moving and handling.
- Treating.

Further reading

Anon. (1996) How To Guides – Pulse Oximetry. *Care Crit Ill* 12(6).

Corne J., Carroll M., Brown I. and Delaney D. (1998) *Chest X-Ray Made Easy*. Churchill Livingstone, Edinburgh.

Jeffries A., Turley A. (1999) *Crash Course Respiratory System*. Horton-Sszar D. (ed). Mosby International Ltd, London.

Ruppel G.L. (1997) Spirometry. *Respir Care Clin N Am* 3(2): 155–181.

Szaflarski N.L. and Cohen N.H. (1991) Use of capnography in critically ill adults. *Heart Lung* 20: 363–374.

Welch J. (2000) Using assessment to identify and prevent critical illness. *Nursing Times Plus* 96(20): 3–4.

Williams A.J. (1998) ABC of oxygen: assessing and interpreting arterial blood gases and acid–base balance. *BMJ* 317(7167): 1213–1216.

Section 2

PATHOPHYSIOLOGY

ACID–BASE BALANCE DISTURBANCES

Description

The body aims to constantly maintain a balance between the production and excretion of acid and alkaline (or base) substances as cells can only function within tight pH limits. If an acid–base balance disturbance occurs, a compensation strategy is initiated.

Key physiological principles

- An acid is a substance that produces free H^+ ions. The body produces 40–80 mmol H^+/day via: protein/amino acid metabolism, anaerobic metabolism and aerobic metabolism producing 20 000 mmol of CO_2/day.

  CO_2 is an acid that can be rapidly excreted by the lungs.

- A buffer is a substance that will 'mop up' excess H^+ ions e.g. hemoglobin, bicarbonate, proteins and phosphates. The most important buffer system is the bicarbonate (HCO_3^-) buffer system.

Bicarbonate buffer system

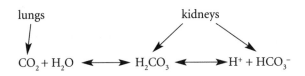

HCO_3^- is an alkaline substance that is excreted slowly by the kidneys.

Table 1. Primary acid–base disturbance shown in bold print with the compensatory mechanism in italic.

	Respiratory acidosis (acute)	Respiratory acidosis (chronic)	Respiratory alkalosis	Metabolic acidosis	Metabolic alkalosis
pH	Decreased	Normal, slight decrease	Increased	Decreased	Increased
P_aCO_2	**Increased**	**Increased**	**Decreased**	*Decreased*	*Slight increase*
HCO_3	*Increased (slight)*	*Increased*	*Decreased*	**Decreased**	**Increased**
Base excess	+ve	+ve	−ve	−ve	+ve

Clinical relevance

Respiratory acidosis

Always secondary to hypoventilation, e.g.:

- airway obstruction, e.g. CAL, bronchospasm/asthma;
- depression of respiratory center, e.g. drugs (sedation, opiates, anesthetic agents), cerebral trauma, space-occupying lesion;
- pulmonary disease, e.g. pulmonary fibrosis, respiratory distress syndrome;
- extrapulmonary thoracic disease, e.g. severe kyphoscoliosis, rib injuries, fractures, flail chest;
- neuromuscular disorders, e.g. poliomyelitis, Guillain–Barré syndrome, muscle relaxants, motor neuron disease, muscular dystrophies (c.f. impaired gaseous exchange).

Respiratory alkalosis

Secondary to:

- hypoxia, e.g. pulmonary disease (pulmonary embolus), pulmonary edema, severe anemia, high altitude;
- increased respiratory drive, e.g. respiratory stimulants (salicylates), cerebral disturbance (infection, trauma, tumor), hyperventilation;
- mechanical overventilation.

Metabolic acidosis

Secondary to:

- increased H^+ formation, e.g. ketoacidosis, lactic acidosis (hypotension, hypoxia, sepsis), poisoning (ethanol, salicylate, ethylene glycol);
- decreased H^+ excretion, e.g. generalized renal failure, renal tubular acidosis;
- loss of bicarbonate, e.g. diarrhea, pancreatic, intestinal and biliary drainage;
- acid ingestion, e.g. acid poisoning, excessive administration of amino acids (lysine, arginine), histamine.

Metabolic alkalosis

Secondary to:

- loss of H^+ via the GI tract: gastric aspiration, vomiting with pyloric obstruction or via the renal system: diuretic therapy (non K^+ sparing);
- rapid correction of chronically raised PCO_2;
- potassium depletion e.g. Cushing's, Crohn's;
- administration of alkali, e.g. inappropriate treatment of acidic states, alkali ingestion.

Oxygen

P_aO_2 is a measure of how much oxygen is dissolved in the plasma but the vast majority of oxygen is bound to Hb. Therefore, anemia and abnormal hemoglobin affect this measurement. However, oxygen levels have no effect on acidity or alkalinity.

Related topics

ACBT +/− manual techniques (p. 71); CPAP (p. 76); IPPB (p. 99); Manual hyperinflation/suction (p. 102); Mechanical ventilation/NIPPV (p. 109); Mobilization (p. 113).

References and further reading

Coleman N.J. (1999) Evaluating arterial blood gas results. *Aust Nurs J* 6(11): suppl 1–3.

Rose B.D. (1994) *Clinical physiology of acid–base and electrolyte disorders.* 4th edition. McGraw-Hill, New York.

Williams A.J. (1998) ABC of oxygen: assessing and interpreting arterial blood gases and acid–base balance. *BMJ* 317(7167): 1213–1216.

AIRFLOW LIMITATION

Description

Airflow limitation occurs as a result of increased airway resistance. The influence of airflow limitation on alveolar ventilation is dependent upon the extent of the resistance.

Key physiological principles

Airway resistance may be increased by:

- Material within the airway lumen, e.g. narrowed or encrusted endotracheal/tracheostomy tubes, mucus, pulmonary edema, foreign bodies, and tumor.
- Contraction, thickening or remodeling of the airway, e.g. bronchial hyper-reactivity, stenosis.
- Extralumenal factors, e.g. compression outside the airway (tumor), airway narrowing secondary to the loss of normal radial traction (emphysema) or airway closure resulting from reduced lung volume.
- In normal lung, a flow-limiting mechanism occurs during forced expiratory maneuvers, termed 'dynamic compression'. Changes in the balance between intrathoracic and airway pressures produce a tendency to airway closure or compression. This effect is not usually seen during *normal* expiration as the retractive force of the lung parenchyma prevents it.
- Resistance to airflow is inversely proportional to lung volume, i.e. resistance is increased with reduced lung volume (c.f. reduced lung volumes).
- Within the bronchial tree, the medium-sized bronchi constitute the principal source of resistance.

Clinical relevance

- Increased resistance to airflow increases the individual's work of breathing and consequently may produce the sensation of dyspnea.
- Presenting signs may include wheeze, tachypnea, impaired exercise tolerance, paradoxical movement of the chest and abdomen, and accessory muscle use.
- Pulmonary function test, in particular PEFR, FEV_1/FVC and flow volume loops, will indicate an obstructive defect.
- When airway resistance is increased, the lung parenchyma diseased, or lung volume reduced, the supporting retractive force of the lung parenchyma is more easily overcome, resulting in marked dynamic compression and gas trapping during forced expiration. In severe lung disease, dynamic compression may even occur during normal expiration. In such situations, the patient may adopt a 'pursed lip' breathing pattern in order to increase airway pressure and improve expiratory airflow.
- The term 'chronic airflow limitation' (CAL) is used to represent three conditions which may co-exist: chronic bronchitis, emphysema and asthma.

- In patients with CAL the lungs frequently become hyperinflated. This may represent an attempt to overcome the resistance to flow, as airway conductance (the reciprocal of resistance) increases with augmented lung volume.
- Lung hyperinflation may also be the result of gas trapping, i.e. reduced lung emptying during expiration secondary to airflow resistance and/or loss of elastic recoil.
- Hyperinflation is associated with adverse effects, e.g. development of intrinsic PEEP producing a consequential increase in the work of breathing, reduced lung compliance and a mechanical disadvantage to respiratory muscle performance.
- In patients with asthma, the airflow limitation may be attributed to any combination of the following factors: mucosal edema ± remodeling, bronchospasm and sputum retention (c.f. inflammation).
- Management of airflow limitation aims where possible to reverse or remove the cause of the increased airway resistance, e.g. pharmacological agents (bronchodilator and anti-inflammatory agents, diuretic agents), invasive procedures (surgery, bronchoscopy), physiotherapy (secretion removal).
- In addition to secretion removal, physiotherapy management should aim to address associated symptoms such as dyspnea and reduced exercise tolerance (e.g. breathing control, activity modification, pulmonary rehabilitation, Buteyko technique).
- Physiotherapy techniques must be applied in a manner that ensures airflow limitation is not further exacerbated, e.g. use of FET.
- In susceptible patients it may be advisable to administer bronchodilator drugs prior to physiotherapy intervention. The physiotherapist should assess that the correct delivery device and administration techniques are used.
- Expiratory wheeze is a common sign in airflow limitation. As the extent of airflow limitation progresses, wheeze may also be heard on inspiration. In extreme cases, when airflow is maximally limited, the chest may be near silent on auscultation.

Related topics

ACBT (p. 71); CPAP (p. 76); Exercise training (p. 79); Inflammation (p. 53); IPPB (p. 99); Mobilization (p. 113).

References and further reading

BTS guidelines for the management of chronic obstructive pulmonary disease: The COPD Guideline Group of the Standards of Care Committee of the BTS (1997). *Thorax* 52(suppl 5): S1–S28.
BTS guidelines on asthma management: 1995 review and position statement (1997). *Thorax* 52: Suppl.
McCarren B. (1992) Dynamic pulmonary hyperinflation. *Aust J Physio* 38(3): 175–179.
Stockley R.A. (2000) New approaches to the management of COPD. *Chest* 117(2 Suppl): 58S–62S.
West J.B. (1995) *Pulmonary Pathophysiology*. 5th edition. Williams and Wilkins, Baltimore.

West J.B. (2000) *Respiratory Physiology – The Essentials*. 6th edition. Lippincott, Williams and Wilkins, Philadelphia.

West J.B. (2001) *Pulmonary Physiology and Pathophysiology – An Integrated, Case-Based Approach*. Lippincott, Williams and Wilkins, Philadelphia.

ALTERED RESPIRATORY COMPLIANCE

Description

Respiratory system compliance describes the relationship between lung volume and the pressure required to generate that volume. It consists of two distinct components: compliance of the chest wall (including the abdomen) and compliance of the lung. Although each component can be measured individually, in clinical practice the clinician is generally concerned with total respiratory system compliance.

Key physiological principles

- The relationship between pressure and volume (and therefore compliance) is demonstrated by the pressure volume curve. A typical compliance curve is shown in Figure 1.

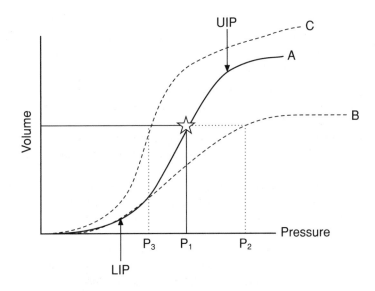

Figure 1. Schematic representation of the relation between pressure and volume. The normal PV curve is represented by curve A. Pressure P_1 is required to generate a specific volume denoted by ☆. If respiratory system compliance decreases (curve B), then a greater pressure (P_2) is required to generate the same volume, i.e. less distensible. If respiratory system compliance increases (curve C), then a lower pressure (P_3) is required to generate the same volume, i.e. more distensible. UIP: upper inflection point represents the beginning of overdistention of lung units. LIP: lower inflection point is thought to represent recruitment of lung units.

- Normal compliance is maintained by regular respiratory cycling with an effective tidal volume.
- Surfactant is an important determinant of compliance. The lipoprotein mixture secreted by alveolar epithelial cells reduces the surface tension in the alveoli and therefore increases the compliance of the lung.
- Surfactant also stabilizes the alveoli protecting against collapse and the transudation of fluid from the capillaries.
- A reduction in respiratory compliance is associated with an increase in work of breathing as a greater pressure change, i.e. inspiratory effort is necessary for the same change in volume (Figure 1).
- The pressure–volume curve of the lung represents the average curve for all lung units. However, within the lung there will be lung units lying at different points on the compliance curve.
- Under normal conditions, areas of dependent lung lie on the steep portion of the pressure volume curve and therefore expand well, whereas areas of nondependent lung lie towards the UIP on the flatter part of the curve and expand less well.
- At low lung volumes this situation may be reversed. Now the nondependent areas are on the steep part of the curve and expand well, whereas the more dependent regions are at or below the LIP and expand poorly, for any given change in pressure (c.f. positioning to improve lung volume).

Clinical relevance

Reduced compliance may be observed in several situations:

- Low lung volume, e.g. postoperatively, postural, obesity.
- Pulmonary venous congestion, interstitial edema and/or fibrosis, e.g. adult respiratory distress syndrome, occupational lung disease.
- Chest wall deformity/injury restricting thoracic expansion, lung consolidation, pleural effusions, pneumothorax, or surfactant dysfunction (e.g. infantile respiratory distress syndrome).
- Conditions characterized by a reduction in compliance are commonly referred to as 'restrictive' in nature (c.f. Assessment tools – spirometry).
- Increased compliance is seen in emphysema, where pulmonary destruction results in loss of retractive forces.
- Recent developments in mechanical ventilation in patients with ALI/ARDS have been influenced by analysis of the PV curve. Results show increased survival in this patient group (Slutsky & Ranieri 2000).
- Pressure-limited ventilation aims to prevent overdistention in more compliant (typically nondependent) regions (c.f. mechanical ventilation, NIPPV).
- The application of PEEP aims to keep less compliant (typically dependent) regions above the LIP, thus 'recruiting' lung volume.
- The use of PEEP avoids the cyclic opening and closing of lung units that is believed to occur around the LIP. This may further reduce injury/trauma associated with mechanical ventilation.
- Physiotherapy techniques which increase FRC, may improve lung compliance

in those patients with low lung volume if a position on the higher part of the PV curve can be maintained (c.f. CPAP, positioning to improve lung volume).

- In patients with reduced chest wall compliance, physiotherapy techniques aimed at improving chest wall mobility, increasing soft tissue extensibility, and strengthening postural muscles may be of benefit (c.f. thoracic mobilization, exercise training)
- The physiotherapist should be aware that patients with reduced respiratory compliance might be vulnerable to the development of respiratory failure secondary to increased respiratory load (c.f. respiratory failure).

Related topics

CPAP (p. 76); Manual hyperinflation (p. 102); Mechanical ventilation (p. 109); NIPPV (p. 118); Positioning to improve lung volume (p. 133); Thoracic mobilization (p. 143).

References and further reading

Slutsky A.S. and Ranieri V.M. (2000) Mechanical ventilation: Lessons from the ARDSNet trial. *Respir Res* 1(2): 73–77.

West J.B. (1995) *Pulmonary Pathophysiology*. 5th edition. Williams and Wilkins, Baltimore.

West J.B. (2000) *Respiratory Physiology – The Essentials*. 6th edition. Lippincott, Williams and Wilkins, Philadelphia.

CHEST WALL DEFORMITY OR DISRUPTION

Description

Collectively, the sternum, thoracic vertebrae, 12 pairs of ribs and the interposing intercostal muscles form the outer chest wall. The chest wall plays a multiple role in maintaining effective ventilation. Any disruption to the chest wall may lead to mechanical dysfunction and inefficient ventilation.

For the purposes of this section 'chest wall' will refer to both pleural and bony components. Respiratory muscle dysfunction is dealt with elsewhere.

Key physiological principles

- The chest wall contributes to total respiratory compliance. Therefore, stiffening of any of the chest wall articulations will result in reduced distensibility of the thorax and lungs.
- Under normal conditions, the bony components of the chest wall provide inherent mechanical stability for the respiratory pump and offer origin and insertion points for respiratory muscles.
- The pleura are a double-layered membrane lining the thoracic cavity. The outermost layer (parietal) is adherent to the chest wall, while the innermost (visceral) is adherent to the outer surface of the lungs. Both the visceral and parietal pleura have direct communications with the lymphatic system.
- Under normal circumstances the pleural cavity, i.e. that separating the visceral and parietal pleura, is a potential space.
- The pressure within the pleural cavity (intrapleural pressure) is normally negative relative to alveolar pressure. This is due to the opposing forces of the lungs (tendency to contract) and the chest wall (tendency to expand). In the absence of this negative pressure, the elastic recoil of the lungs would dominate and the lungs would collapse.
- Intrapleural pressure becomes more negative from nondependent to dependent regions, due to the increasing weight of the lung. It is this intrapleural pressure gradient which influences the normal distribution of gas.

Clinical relevance

Pleural disruption

- In certain situations the pleural cavity may be disrupted and the 'potential' space becomes an 'actual' space. This may be a result of air (pneumothorax), transudate/exudate (effusion), chyle (chylothorax), blood (hemothorax) or pus (empyema) in the pleural cavity.
- Consequent alteration in the intrapleural pressure will cause the underlying lung to collapse. Insertion of an intercostal drain or surgery (e.g. decortication, pleurectomy) may be indicated.

- Pneumothoraces may result from rupture of an air-filled bleb on the lung surface, from thoracic trauma, or secondary to high intrathoracic pressures. Physiotherapy techniques involving application of positive pressure are contraindicated in the *absence* of a patent intercostal drain (c.f. IPPB, CPAP, manual hyperinflation).
- Pleural effusions occur when fluid forms faster than it can be removed. Causative factors may be:
  - increased capillary permeability, e.g. inflammatory conditions such as infection or rheumatoid disease;
  - increased capillary pressure, e.g. congestive cardiac failure;
  - decreased colloid osmotic pressure, e.g. low albumin associated with malnourishment;
  - increased negative intrapleural pressure, e.g. atelectasis;
  - impaired lymphatic drainage, e.g. mediastinal tumor.
- In the presence of significant effusion, lung volume cannot be restored until the effusion is drained. The insertion of a 'pig tail' catheter or chest drain may be required.

Chest wall disorders

- Chest wall disorders, e.g. kyphoscoliosis, thoracoplasty, circumferential burns/scarring, ankylosing spondylitis, may result in a dramatic reduction in respiratory compliance and increased work of breathing (c.f. NIPPV).
- Respiratory muscles may also be placed at a mechanical disadvantage due to altered length–tension relationships and fiber alignment (c.f. respiratory muscle dysfunction).
- Depending upon severity of the chest wall disorder, patients may be predisposed to persistent atelectasis and chronic respiratory failure. NIPPV may be indicated, particularly in those patients presenting with nocturnal hypoventilation and/or hypercapnia (c.f. NIPPV).
- Exercise training/pulmonary rehabilitation may be of benefit in patients with chest wall disorders to maintain or improve exercise tolerance by improving efficiency of oxygen utilization at muscle level (c.f. exercise training – 1, exercise training in pulmonary rehabilitation).
- Chronic respiratory disease in itself may predispose to chest wall problems. Patients commonly present with stiffness and postural abnormalities. The physiotherapist should insure that these problems are prevented where possible, and treated where they have already developed (c.f. thoracic mobilization)

Disruption of the ribs

- Chest trauma may be associated with disruption of both the pleura (pneumothorax) and the chest wall (rib fractures).
- Rib fractures may occur in the absence of trauma, e.g. pathological fractures or with only minimal force, e.g. osteoporotic individuals.
- Even simple rib fractures can cause extreme pain. Analgesia is the key element of management, allowing mobilization, effective deep breathing and supported coughing. Appropriately managed, respiratory complications such as atelectasis

or pulmonary infection may be minimized. Prior to discharge it is advisable to educate the patient in continuing management of pain, respiratory function and postural correction (c.f. pain management).

- Multiple rib fractures (more than 2–3 ribs fractured in two places) result in a flail segment, whereby the affected part of the chest moves paradoxically due to instability. This constitutes a significant injury and is often associated with underlying lung contusion.

- Lung contusion is the result of bleeding and edema and often appears radiologically 12–24 hours after the injury. Contusion may be present in the absence of rib fractures. The reduction in alveolar ventilation may produce a marked mismatch between ventilation and perfusion. CPAP or mechanical ventilation may be necessary (c.f. impaired gaseous exchange, CPAP, mechanical ventilation).

- Rib fractures may often be missed radiologically. Clinical diagnosis, e.g. nature of injury, pain particularly on inspiration and crepitus is often of value.

Related topics

CPAP (p. 76); Exercise training – 1 (p. 79); Exercise training in pulmonary rehabilitation (p. 85); Mechanical ventilation (p. 109); NIPPV (p. 118); Thoracic mobilization (p. 143).

References and further reading

Pozzi E. and Gulotta C. (1993) Classification of chest wall diseases. *Monaldi Arch Chest Dis* **48**(1): 65–68.
Sahn S. (1988) State of the art. The pleura. *Am Rev Respir Dis* **138**(1): 184–234.
West J.B. (1995) *Pulmonary Pathophysiology*. 5th edition. Williams and Wilkins, Baltimore.

CONTROL OF BREATHING

Description

Breathing takes place secondary to the contraction and relaxation of the respiratory muscles, which occurs automatically without conscious effort. This action is dependent on an intact nervous system relaying impulses from the rhythm generator and the respiratory centers in the brainstem, via the spinal cord and phrenic nerve to the muscles of respiration.

- Breathing is constantly adjusted to match changes in metabolic demands, e.g. increased metabolism, exercise or breathing at altitude.
- How effective an adaptive change in breathing pattern is, will depend on the mechanical properties of the thorax and the efficiency of gas exchange by the lungs.
- Breathing is regularly modified to accommodate many activities, e.g. speech, voluntary movement and exercise, swallowing and coughing.
- Breathing pattern can be influenced by voluntary cortical control during wakefulness.
- Various diseases and pharmacological agents can influence the control of breathing.

Key physiological principles

- The regulation of breathing is dependent on constant feedback to the respiratory centers from several different receptors.
- Receptors sensitive to mechanical stimulation are sited in the airways (stretch and irritant), around the alveoli (juxta receptors) and in the chest wall (Golgi tendon organs and muscle spindles).
- Chemical stimuli such as PO_2, PCO_2 and pH can dramatically influence the control of breathing.
- The peripheral chemoreceptors are sited in the aorta (aortic bodies) and the common carotid artery (carotid bodies). These receptors are stimulated by a decrease of arterial PO_2, a decrease in arterial pH and respiratory oscillations of PCO_2 (Dutton *et al.* 1968).
- The peripheral chemoreceptors can also be stimulated by hypoperfusion, possibly secondary to 'stagnant hypoxia'. Clinically this may occur during prolonged hypotension.
- An elevated blood temperature will stimulate breathing via the peripheral chemoreceptors.
- Various drugs and other chemical stimulants influence breathing via the peripheral chemoreceptors, e.g. nicotine, aceytlcholine, cyanide and carbon monoxide.
- The central chemoreceptors are sited on the anterolateral surface of the medulla in the brainstem. These receptors are stimulated by a rise in PCO_2, which produces an equal rise in CSF, cerebral tissue, and jugular venous PCO_2.
- Segmental and intersegmental reflexes at a spinal cord level may also affect breathing.

- Baroreceptors, primarily associated with arterial blood pressure regulation can influence breathing pattern. A fall in BP leads to hyperventilation, while a rise in BP produces hypoventilation and ultimately apnea (Heymans & Neil 1958).

Clinical relevance

- At sleep onset, loss of the wakefulness drive to breath is associated with a change in breathing pattern. A reduction in tidal volume (V_T) rather than a change in respiratory frequency results in a fall in minute ventilation (Douglas *et al.* 1982).
- Sleep is associated with several disordered breathing patterns. Central sleep apnea occurs secondary to a loss of the central drive to breath during sleep. In some patient groups this is thought to be due to reduced levels of arterial CO_2.
- Cheyne–Stokes respiration (CSR) is the most common form of sleep disordered breathing seen in 40–50% of patients with CHF (Javaheri *et al.* 1995).
- This periodic breathing pattern is characterized by periods of central apnea or hypopnea alternating with a crescendo–decrescendo fluctuation in tidal volume (Harrison *et al.* 1934).
- CSR is also seen in patients with a severe neurological insult. In the end stage of both CHF and some neurological diseases CSR is also seen during wakefulness.
- The presence of several respiratory centers has been established from animal models, e.g. inspiratory, expiratory, apneustic and pneumotaxic. Pathological abnormalities in these specific sites have elicited specific breathing patterns associated with these respiratory centers.
- The sensation of breathlessness or dyspnea is the subjective awareness of discomfort related to breathing. Many physiological and psychological factors are likely to contribute to this sensation. Consequently, the principles of management are also multifactorial (Joffe & Berend 1997).
- Hyperventilation constitutes breathing in excess of metabolic requirements, and can occur for a variety of organic or physiological reasons, e.g. secondary to poisoning (salicylates or ethyl alcohol), or to induce a compensatory respiratory alkalosis in the presence of a metabolic acidosis.
- Hyperventilation syndrome or chronic hyperventilation can occur in response to both psychological and physiological stimuli or without a known etiology (Gardner & Bass 1989). Panic attacks, anxiety and phobias may be associated with this syndrome.
- The use of breathing control, relaxation, anxiety management and positioning may be beneficial in relieving the symptoms of hyperventilation syndrome (c.f. ACBT, positioning to relieve breathlessness).
- Neurophysiological facilitation of respiration techniques has also been used successfully in the treatment of hyperventilation syndrome (c.f. NPF).

Related topics

Breathing control in ACBT (p. 71); CPAP (p. 76); NIPPV (p. 118); NPF (p. 115); Positioning to relieve breathlessness (p. 131).

References and further reading

Douglas N.J., White D.P., Pickett C.K., Weil J.V. and Zwillich C.W. (1982) Respiration during sleep in normal man. *Thorax* **37**: 840–844.

Dutton R.E., Fitzgerald R.S. and Gross N. (1968) Ventilatory response to square-wave forcing of carbon dioxide at the carotid bodies. *Resp Physiol* **4**: 101.

Gardner W.N. and Bass C. (1989). Hyperventilation in clinical practice. *Br J Hosp Med* **41**(1): 73–81.

Folgering H. (1999) The pathophysiology of hyperventilation syndrome. *Monaldi Arch Chest Dis* **54**(4): 365–372.

Harrison T., King C. and Calhoun J. (1934) Congestive heart failure. Cheyne–Stokes respiration as a cause of paroxysmal nocturnal dyspnoea at the onset of sleep. *Arch Int Med* **53**: 891–910.

Heymans C. and Neil E. (1958) *Reflexogenic Areas of the Cardiovascular System.* Boston, Mass, Little Brown; London, Churchill.

Javaheri S., Parker T.J., Wexler L., Michaels S.E., Stanberry E., Nishyama H. and Roselle G.A. (1995) Occult sleep-disordered breathing in stable congestive heart failure. *Ann Intern Med* **122**: 487–492.

Joffe D. and Berend N. (1997) Assessment and management of dyspnoea. *Respirology* **2**(1): 33–43.

Thomas M., McKinley R.K., Freeman E., Foy C. (2001) Prevalance of dysfunctional breathing in patients treated for asthma in primary care: cross sectional study. *BMJ* **322**(7294): 1098–1100.

DECONDITIONING

Description

Multisystem deconditioning affecting cardiovascular, respiratory and neuromusculoskeletal systems may occur as a result of restricted physical activity, and reduces the ability to perform work.

Key physiological principles

- The extent of deconditioning is influenced by many factors including age, pre-morbid condition, nature of the illness/injury, nutrition, drug management, level or nature of immobility, duration of immobility.
- Physiological changes are associated with immobility/reduced mobility, whether iatrogenic (e.g. sedated, paralysed and ventilated patient) or secondary to trauma or disease (e.g. CAL, angina, intermittent claudication).

Effects on the cardiovascular system

- Reduced maximal stroke volume.
- Reduced cardiac output.
- Reduced oxygen uptake.
- Decreased orthostatic tolerance → postural hypotension.
- Predisposition to thromboembolism during period of immobility (increased blood viscosity and vascular stasis).

Effects on the respiratory system

- Adverse effects on FRC, compliance, resistance and closing capacity when associated with supine position.
- Predisposition to respiratory complications during period of immobilization.

Effects on the neuromusculoskeletal system

- Increased muscle fatigue associated with reduced muscle blood flow, capillarization and oxidative enzymes.
- Loss of muscle mass with a reduction in strength.
- Contractures may occur due to muscle shortening or changes in peri/intra-articular connective tissue.
- Decreased bone mineral density.

Clinical relevance

- An holistic approach to patient management is essential in order to address factors which compound the deconditioning process, e.g. use of paralysing

agents, malnutrition, electrolyte imbalance, anxiety, co-existing disease. For best results, the patient's condition should be optimized.
- Specific exercise modalities should be applied to maintain aerobic capacity and prevent neuro-musculoskeletal deterioration both during/after a period of reduced physical activity and in the presence of disease associated with reduced physical activity (c.f. exercise training)
- Deconditioning invariably results in impaired functional independence, and a higher risk of falls and injury.
- Preventing or minimizing the effects of deconditioning has both cost and quality implications for the healthcare system and the patient.

Related topics

ACBT (p. 71); IPPB (p. 99); Exercise training (p. 79); Mobilization (p. 113); Thoracic mobilization (p. 143).

References and further reading

Convertino V.A., Bloomfield S.A. and Greenleaf J.E. (1995) An overview of the issues: physiological effects of bed rest and restricted physical activity. *Med Sci Sport Ex* **29**(2): 187–190.

DISORDERS OF THE PULMONARY CIRCULATION 1 – PULMONARY EDEMA

Description

The accumulation of fluid in the extracellular spaces of the lung parenchyma. This process can occur as a complication of a number of diseases of the heart and lungs.

- There are two stages in the formation of pulmonary edema.
- Firstly, the formation of interstitial edema, i.e. engorgement of the perivascular and peribronchial interstitial tissue.
- Secondly, the presence of alveolar edema where fluid has passed into and filled successive alveoli.

Key physiological principles

- Under normal conditions, the pulmonary capillary endothelium is highly permeable to water and various solutes, but not to plasma proteins.
- The alveolar epithelium is less permeable to water and solutes, keeping the alveoli free of excess fluid.
- The movement of fluid across the endothelium is dependent on the balance between the hydrostatic pressure, which tends to move fluid out of the capillary and into the interstitial space, and the plasma oncotic pressure, which tends to hold fluid in the intravascular space.
- Once fluid has left the capillary and has entered the interstitial space of the alveolar wall, it tracks to the perivascular and peribronchial interstitium. Here, some fluid is removed via the lymphatic system while some continues to move through loose interstitial tissue.
- The net movement of fluid is governed by Starling's equation;

$$Q = [(P_c - P_i) - \sigma(\pi_c - \pi_i)]$$

where Q = net flow out of capillary,
P_c/P_i = hydrostatic pressure in capillary/interstitium,
π_c/π_i = colloid oncotic pressure in capillary/interstitium.

- A decrease in plasma oncotic pressure, increase in hydrostatic pressure, increase in endothelial/alveolar membrane permeability or decrease in lymphatic clearance, will lead to the development of pulmonary edema.

Clinical relevance

- Pulmonary edema can occur secondary to a variety of conditions.
- Increased pulmonary capillary hydrostatic pressure most commonly causes pulmonary edema. This may be seen in heart disease secondary to an increased left atrial pressure, e.g. acute MI, hypertensive left ventricular failure and mitral

valve disease (c.f. heart failure). Fluid overloading following an intravenous infusion can also raise capillary pressure and may lead to pulmonary edema.

- Increased pulmonary capillary permeability may occur secondary to the inhalation of toxic substances, e.g. chlorine or sulfur dioxide, or via circulating endotoxin. Increased capillary permeability is seen in adult respiratory distress syndrome/acute lung injury, sepsis and systemic inflammatory response syndrome (c.f. infection and inflammation).
- A reduced colloid osmotic pressure may exaggerate pulmonary edema, e.g. hypoalbuminemia in adult respiratory distress syndrome, malnutrition or intravenous fluid overloading with saline.
- Lymphatic obstruction or increased central venous pressure can impair lymphatic drainage.
- Pulmonary edema can occur without specific etiology, e.g. at high altitude, or following trauma to the central nervous system.
- Patients with pulmonary edema complain of dyspnea and adopt a rapid shallow breathing pattern (c.f. positioning to relieve breathlessness).
- During the first stage of perivascular and peribronchial engorgement, a persistent cough often develops which is usually unproductive. However, once alveolar edema is established patients may expectorate pink frothy sputum.

Related topics

CPAP (p. 76); Mechanical ventilation (p. 109); Positioning to relieve breathlessness (p. 131).

References and further reading

Cotter G., Kaluski E., Moshkovitz Y., Milovanov O., Krakover R. and Vered Z. (2001) Pulmonary edema: new insight on pathogenesis and treatment. *Curr Opin Cardiol* **16**(3): 159–163. Review.

Miserocchi G., Negrini D., Passi A. and De Luca G. (2001) Development of lung edema: interstitial fluid dynamics and molecular structure. *News Physiol Sci* **16**: 66-71. Review.

DISORDERS OF THE PULMONARY CIRCULATION 2 – PULMONARY EMBOLISM

Description

Commonly attributable to detached fragments of venous thrombi formed in the deep veins of the lower limbs, which lodge in a branch of the pulmonary artery. Rarely, may also be caused by fat or air emboli.

Key physiological principles

- Several factors may precipitate the formation of a thrombus. Most commonly, prolonged immobilization, direct local pressure or venous obstruction producing stasis of blood.
- Pathological conditions affecting the viscosity of blood, e.g. sickle cell disease or polycythemia, lead to sluggish flow.
- Increased coagulability may occur secondary to pregnancy, surgery, malignancy or the use of oral contraceptives.
- Inflammation or direct trauma may damage the vessel walls producing areas susceptible to clot adherence.

Clinical relevance

- Pleuritic pain and dyspnea often accompany a pulmonary embolus (c.f. positioning to relieve breathlessness, physiotherapy management of pain).
- Effective analgesia should be administered to prevent hypoventilation (c.f. impaired gaseous exchange).
- Patients may have a productive cough and expectorate blood-stained secretions.
- A pleural rub may be heard on auscultation (c.f. assessment tools).
- Pulmonary emboli may lead to the infarction of lung parenchyma supplied by that vessel.
- Hemorrhage and atelectasis may occur at the site of infarction.
- Interruption of lung perfusion, and associated inflammation leads to V/Q mismatching and hypoxia (c.f. impaired gaseous exchange).
- Massive emboli may produce hemodynamic collapse, shock, chest pain and a loss of consciousness.

Related topics

Physiotherapy management of pain (p. 126); Positioning to relieve breathlessness (p. 131).

References and further reading

Riedel M. (2001) Acute pulmonary embolism 1: pathophysiology, clinical presentation, and diagnosis. *Heart* **85**(2): 229–240. Review.
Riedel M. (2001) Acute pulmonary embolism 2: treatment. *Heart* **85**(3): 351–360. Review.

DISORDERS OF THE PULMONARY CIRCULATION 3 – PULMONARY HYPERTENSION

Description

Pulmonary hypertension is defined as a mean pulmonary artery pressure > 3.3 kPa (25 mmHg) at rest or 4.0 kPa (30 mmHg) on exercise.

Key physiological principles

- Three mechanisms may lead to the development of pulmonary hypertension.
- An increased left atrial pressure, e.g. secondary to mitral stenosis or left ventricular failure, will lead to pulmonary hypertension via backpressure across the pulmonary veins.
- An increase in pulmonary blood flow beyond the capacitance of the pulmonary vascular bed; this may occur with some congenital heart defects.
- A reduction in the cross-sectional area of the pulmonary vascular bed:
  - vasoconstriction due to hypoxia, e.g. CAL;
  - obstruction of the pulmonary vascular bed, e.g. pulmonary embolus;
  - destruction of the pulmonary vascular bed due to parenchymal lung disorders, e.g. emphysema, pulmonary fibrosis.
- More than one component can occur in a disease state, e.g. in CAL hypoxia and destruction of the pulmonary vascular bed contribute to raised pulmonary artery pressures.
- Pulmonary hypertension in most lung conditions is normally fairly modest (< 45 mmHg), but may be severe in primary pulmonary hypertension and pulmonary hypertension secondary to recurrent thromboembolic disease, where pulmonary artery pressures may reach systemic levels.
- Long-term oxygen therapy (LTOT) (>16 hours/day) may be of benefit in the treatment of pulmonary hypertension in some patients with CAL.
- Contrary to popular belief, cor pulmonale (peripheral edema in the presence of chronic lung disease) is not usually associated with *severe* pulmonary hypertension with subsequent right heart failure. Fluid retention is mainly due to effects of hypoxia and hypercapnia on the kidney.

Clinical relevance

- LTOT may be appropriate in some patients with CAL to prevent progression of pulmonary hypertension (c.f. oxygen therapy).
- Cardiac dysfunction, e.g. arrhythmias, angina, may occur with more severe pulmonary hypertension.

Related topics

Heart failure (p. 41); Oxygen therapy (p. 122); Positioning to relieve breathlessness (p. 131).

References and further reading

Galie N. and Torbicki A. (2001) Pulmonary arterial hypertension: new ideas and perspectives. *Heart* 85(4): 475–480. Review.

Krowka M.J. (2000) Pulmonary hypertension: diagnostics and therapeutics. *Mayo Clin Proc* 75(6): 625–630.

EFFECTS OF GENERAL ANESTHESIA

Description

General anesthesia (GA) is commonly achieved with the use of intravenous and inhaled anesthetic agents. Further drugs may be used to elicit muscle relaxation.

Key physiological principles

- The dose response of an inhaled anesthetic agent is measured by minimum alveolar concentration (MAC). This is the alveolar concentration that allows 50% of patients to move to a given stimuli.
- Certain anesthetic agents affect the central response to hypercapnia. Isofluorane produces marked respiratory depression at 1 MAC.
- Without surgical stimuli, the minute volume may fall to very low levels and a marked hypercapnia may occur. The clinical significance of this hypercapnia is not clear. In the US most patients are mechanically ventilated to prevent this effect.
- Anesthetic agents also cause a dramatic attenuation of the respiratory response to hypoxemia. As little as 0.1 MAC, i.e. recovery room levels, can produce this response.
- Muscle relaxants (acetylcholine antagonists) are used, acting at the neuro-muscular junction to cause paralysis. These drugs alter the function of the respiratory and upper airway muscles, producing a change in the pattern of breathing and predisposing to obstruction.
- Functional residual capacity (FRC) decreases by 16–20% when compared to the awake, supine subject. This response occurs minutes after induction of GA and persists in the early postoperative period. The reduction in FRC has a weak but significant correlation with age.
- The causes of reduced FRC have been proposed: decreased cross-sectional area of the rib cage, cephalad movement of the diaphragm, loss of respiratory muscle tone, gas trapping, blood shift out of the thorax (less splinting of lung parenchyma) (Rehder 1990).
- The effects of a reduced FRC include a reduction in the oxygen reservoir, and reduced compliance predisposing to alveolar collapse (c.f. reduced lung volumes).
- Lung volume decreases during GA, and therefore resistance to flow is increased. However, the bronchodilator effects of volatile anesthetic agents counteract this.
- Alveolar dead space is increased during GA because of preferential ventilation of areas with high ventilation/perfusion (V/Q) ratios. Consequently, V/Q mismatching occurs during GA, with venous admixture elevated by a mean of 10% (c.f. impaired gaseous exchange).
- General anesthesia adversely affects lung mucociliary clearance (Houtmeyers *et al.* 1999) (c.f. impaired tracheobronchial clearance).

Clinical relevance

- Postoperative hypoxemia is a common and frequently prolonged phenomenon. Contributing factors include:
  - residual effects of anesthesia;
  - sleep-disordered breathing;
  - pulmonary complications, e.g. infection, edema, embolus, pneumothorax;
  - altered pattern of breathing secondary to pain or surgical procedure;
  - reduced lung volume (c.f. reduced lung volumes, altered respiratory compliance).
- Postoperative hypoxemia has been implicated in myocardial ischemia and infarction, cerebrovascular accident, impaired wound healing, confusion and death.
- Risk factors associated with increased morbidity and mortality include:
  - increasing age;
  - obesity;
  - history of smoking;
  - pre-existing pulmonary or cardiac pathology.
- Consequently, therapeutic intervention should include appropriate oxygen therapy and oxygen saturation monitoring (c.f. oxygen therapy).

Related topics

ACBT (p. 71); CPAP (p. 76); IPPB (p. 99); Mobilization (p. 113); Oxygen therapy/humidification (p. 122); Positioning to increase lung volume (p. 133).

References and further reading

Brooks-Brunn J.A. (1995) Postoperative atelectasis and pneumonia. *Heart Lung* **24**: 94–115.

Houtmeyers E., Gosselink R., Gayan-Ramirez G. and Decramer M. (1999) Regulation of mucociliary clearance in health and disease. *Euro Respir J* **13**: 1177–1188.

Nunn J.F. (1990) Effects of anaesthesia on respiration. *Br J Anaesth* **65**(1): 54–62.

Rehder K. (1990) Mechanics of the lung and chest wall. *Acta Anaesthesiol Scand* **94**: 32–36.

HEART FAILURE

Description

Heart failure is a clinical syndrome in which impaired cardiac pumping decreases ejection and impedes venous return (Mann *et al.* 1992). Depressed myocardial contractility and relaxation generally further complicate these hemodynamic abnormalities.

- The term 'heart failure' encompasses a whole spectrum of disorders from acute failure (shock states) to congestive heart failure (CHF).
- In many patients, a recognizable pathological condition initiates heart failure, e.g. with myocardial disease, such as cardiomyopathy, infarction or fibrosis, impaired contractility and decreased cardiac output result in dysfunction.
- Systemic arterial hypertension, aortic valve disease or aortic stenosis produce pressure overload of the ventricles, where the ventricle fails to pump adequately against an increased afterload, culminating in left-sided heart failure.
- Pulmonary artery stenosis and pulmonary hypertension produce pressure overload of the right ventricle, precipitating right-sided failure.
- The term CHF refers to the situation where both ventricles have failed. CHF is a condition where the output of the heart is insufficient to meet the demands of the tissues, despite adequate venous filling (Braunwald *et al.* 1997).

Key physiological principles

- CHF should be regarded as a disease not only of the heart, but also of the whole cardiovascular system.
- A series of systemic compensatory and adaptive changes takes place, which initially assists maintenance of cardiac output, but ultimately contributes to the ongoing pathophysiology.
- The first adaptation that occurs in response to hemodynamic overload is hypertrophy of the myocyte. This helps to reduce ventricular wall stress and maintains cardiac pump function in the face of increased afterload or myocyte death. Although initially this is beneficial, over time there is a gradual decline in function.
- A reduced cardiac output may produce a lower systemic blood pressure. Subsequent low renal perfusion pressure initiates a second compensatory mechanism via the endocrine system, by stimulating the renin–angiotensin–aldosterone axis.
- The release of renin provides the catalyst for the conversion of angiotensin II from angiotensin I. Angiotensin II is a potent vasoconstrictor, which acts on the systemic vasculature increasing peripheral vascular resistance. This produces an increase in circulating blood volume in an attempt to facilitate ventricular contraction. However, increased blood volume increases preload on the right side of the heart, ultimately increasing cardiac work and therefore myocardial oxygen demand.
- The release of aldosterone stimulates the retention of salt and water by the

kidney, further increasing circulating volume, which may compound the problem of increased preload.

- Higher centers in the brain are also sensitive to a fall in cardiac output, via high- and low-pressure baroreceptors which stimulate activation of the sympathetic nervous system (SNS). The production of norepinephrine (noradrenaline) is increased, producing both inotropic (strength of contraction) and chronotropic (frequency of contraction) effects on the heart in an attempt to compensate for the reduced cardiac output.
- As SNS stimulation persists epinephrine (adrenaline) is also released. CHF patients who have high plasma noradrenaline levels have a worse prognosis than those patients with levels within a normal range (Jackson *et al.* 2000).
- As the disease process advances, counterbalancing hormones such as atrial natriuretic peptide, brain natriuretic peptide, prostaglandins and dopamine are secreted, which essentially promote diuresis with the inhibition of renal sodium (Na^+) and water reabsorption. Plasma atrial natriuretic peptide levels are increased severalfold in patients with CHF, though its action appears to be relatively insensitive (Omland *et al.* 1995).
- Healthy vascular endothelium secretes both endothelin (vasoconstrictor substance) and nitric oxide (vasodilator substance). The balance of these two substances is deranged in patients with CHF (Wei *et al.* 1994). The increased release of endothelin promotes vasoconstriction rendering the counter-balancing hormones less effective (Lerman *et al.* 1991).

Clinical relevance

- The signs and symptoms of heart failure are manifested as a result of the complications of ventricular dysfunction. Right ventricular failure produces peripheral edema, which when severe can lead to hepatic and renal insufficiency.
- Raised pulmonary venous pressure, a product of left ventricular failure, produces pulmonary congestion, which impairs gaseous exchange and causes the symptom of breathlessness (c.f. pulmonary edema).
- The beneficial adaptations and compensatory mechanisms, which are evoked throughout the process of heart failure, ultimately become decompensatory and pathological, increasing myocardial oxygen demand and imposing a greater work load on the failing heart.
- The failure of either or both ventricles leads to a reduction in cardiac output, and consequently the patient often complains of fatigue and a reduced exercise capacity (c.f. exercise training – 1, exercise training in cardiac rehabilitation).
- Peripheral edema and breathlessness lead to difficulty in mobilization.
- Breathing control may be of benefit to assist mobilization and stair climbing (c.f. ACBT)
- CHF patients may have increased symptoms when supine and often present with paroxysmal nocturnal dyspnea.
- Patients with CHF may develop sleep-disordered breathing, leading to sleep disruption, daytime somnolence and increased fatigue (c.f. control of breathing).

- CPAP, and bi-level positive pressure devices may offer some symptomatic relief (c.f. CPAP, NIPPV).

Related topics

CPAP (p. 76); Exercise training – 1 (p. 79); Exercise training in cardiac rehabilitation (p. 82); NIPPV (p. 118); Positioning to relieve breathlessness (p. 131).

References and further reading

Braunwald E. and Antman E.M. (1997) Evidence-based coronary care. *Ann Intern Med* **126**(7): 551–553.

Jackson G., Gibbs C.R., Davis R.C. and Lip G.Y.H. (2000) ABC of heart failure: Pathophysiology. *BMJ* **320**: 167–169.

Lerman A., Hildebrand F.L.J., Aarhus L.L. and Burnett J.C.J. (1991) Endothelin had biological actions at pathophysiological concentrations. *Circulation* **83**: 1808–1814.

Mann D.L., Kent R., Parson B., et al. (1992) Adrenergic effects on the biology of the adult mammalian cardiocyte. *Circulation* **85**: 790–804.

Omland T., Bonarjee V.V. and Caidahl K. (1995) Neurohumoral measurements as indicators of long-term prognosis after acute myocardial infarction. *Am J Cardiol* **76**: 230–235.

Wei C.M., Lerman A. and Rodeheffer R.J.E. (1994) Endothelin in human congestive heart failure. *Circulation* **89**: 1580–1586.

IMPAIRED GASEOUS EXCHANGE

Description

The term hypoxia refers to inadequate oxygen delivery to the tissues to meet the prevailing metabolic demands. Hypoxia can be due to reduced arterial oxygen content (e.g. anemia), reduced tissue blood flow, or reduced arterial saturation (hypoxemia). Hypoxemia can result from a lower inspired oxygen concentration (e.g. altitude), from a reduction in alveolar ventilation (hypoventilation), from diffusion impairments (e.g. interstitial lung disease) or from inequalities in the relationship between alveolar ventilation and blood flow (ventilation–perfusion mismatch).

Key physiological principles

- The movement of oxygen from the atmosphere to its ultimate site of utilization in the body's cells involves many different processes. Movement through the airways takes place by convection and diffusion.
- Diffusion is then the main transport mechanism across the alveolar–capillary membrane through the plasma to the red blood cell, where oxygen combines with hemoglobin.
- Blood travels through the arterial system to the small capillaries where oxygen, once unloaded in the tissues, diffuses across the cell to reach the mitochondria.

Inspired oxygen concentration

- The partial pressure of inspired oxygen (P_iO_2) is calculated using the following equation:

  (barometric pressure − partial pressure of water vapour 47 mmHg) × 0.2093.

  Barometric pressure decreases with distance above the earth's surface in an exponential relationship. Therefore the PO_2 of inspired gas at sea level is 110 mmHg whereas at 3000 m the PO_2 is only 55 mmHg.
- Therefore, the hypoxemia associated with breathing at altitude is produced by a reduced concentration of oxygen present in the inspired air.

Hypoventilation

- For the process of cellular respiration to continue effectively, oxygen is removed from alveolar blood for utilization in the tissues, and CO_2 is excreted. This process is dependent on adequate ventilation by the lungs, to replenish alveolar oxygen with fresh breath drawn in from the atmosphere, whilst CO_2 is expelled.
- If total ventilation is reduced and does not match the rate of oxygen consumption (and CO_2 production) then the effective O_2 in the alveolus will fall, and arterial hypoxemia will occur (Weinberger *et al.* 1989). This situation is called hypoventilation. Hypoventilation is always associated with hypercapnia.

$$PCO_2 = \frac{VCO_2}{VA} \times K$$

i.e.: if alveolar ventilation is halved then PCO_2 is doubled.

- Hypoventilation may occur secondary to airway obstruction, depression of the respiratory center, pulmonary disease, extrathoracic disease or neuromuscular disease (c.f. acid–base disturbances).

Impaired diffusion

- If the diffusion pathway between alveolar gas to pulmonary capillary blood is impaired, PO_2 equlibration may not have time to occur.
- Under normal conditions, there is a significant amount of 'reserve' time for this process to take place.
- However, if the alveolar–capillary membrane is significantly affected, diffusion impairment may produce hypoxemia, particularly on exercise.

Ventilation–perfusion mismatch

- To ensure adequate transfer of both O_2 and CO_2 the body depends on the 'matching' of ventilation and blood flow in various regions of the lung.
- An alteration of either ventilation or perfusion will cause an alteration in gas transfer efficiency. This is called a V/Q mismatch.

Clinical relevance

- At altitude when exposed to this reduced level of oxygen the body initiates various responses during a process known as acclimatization. The most rapid response is hyperventilation (Severinghaus et al. 1992), caused by the peripheral chemoreceptors that are stimulated by a reduced P_aO_2. However, the increased respiratory rate is rapidly antagonized by the resultant hypocapnia. With time, this negative feedback loop is nullified by the blood–brain barrier active transport system producing shifts in levels of CSF bicarbonate, which normalizes CSF pH and allows ventilation to increase and further raise PO_2 levels (Michel et al. 1963).
- Arterial blood pH is also returned to normal by renal excretion of bicarbonate ions. Interestingly, natives of high altitude have a significantly reduced ventilatory response to hypoxia.
- Hypoventilation can be drug induced, leading to the depression of the central respiratory center, e.g. morphine or barbiturates.
- Damage or disease of the chest wall or respiratory muscles may also reduce adequate pulmonary minute ventilation, e.g. scoliosis, high spinal injury, poliomyelitis.
- The immediate problem of arterial hypoxemia may be relieved by the use of supplemental oxygen, but this will have little effect on the hypercapnia (c.f.

oxygen therapy). To correct the disturbance completely the respiratory rate and depth must be restored to a level sufficient to give normal alveolar tensions of carbon dioxide and oxygen.

- In medical practice this can be performed by reversal of the cause of hypoventilation (e.g. management of drug overdose), or by the institution of ventilatory support (c.f. mechanical ventilation, NIPPV, IPPB).

- Inequalities in V/Q (mismatching of ventilation and perfusion), result in arterial blood gas derangements: hypoxemia and hypercapnia. The V/Q ratio may be decreased (underventilation of perfused alveoli, e.g. atelectasis), or increased (impaired perfusion of ventilated alveoli, e.g. pulmonary embolus or low output states). These states are often referred to as wasted perfusion (shunt) and wasted ventilation (increased alveolar dead space), respectively.

- If the chemoreceptors respond to the elevated P_aCO_2, alveolar ventilation may be increased. This may be effective in normalizing the P_aCO_2, but is of little consequence in raising P_aO_2.

- Blood from lung units with a normal V/Q ratio will already be fully saturated, and the capacity to further increase oxygen carriage is negligible. Therefore, it cannot compensate for the hypoxemic blood from other lung units. This also explains the relative inadequacy of supplemental oxygen therapy in significant V/Q mismatch (c.f. respiratory failure).

- Ventilation–perfusion imbalance is the main determinant of hypoxemia in respiratory diseases such as CAL, pneumonia, and pulmonary fibrosis (Wagner *et al.* 1991).

- Many factors influence pulmonary vascular tone, and thus the regional distribution of pulmonary blood flow, the most important being the composition of the respiratory gases with both hypoxia and hypercapnia inducing vasoconstriction (Fishman 1961).

- Hypoxic pulmonary vasoconstriction (HPV) is the physiological response that decreases the perfusion to underventilated hypoxic alveoli, thereby optimizing V/Q matching and restoring P_aO_2.

- Loss of HPV has serious implications, and is thought to be the mechanism underlying the development of refractory hypoxemia in pneumonia or following acute lung injury (Barnes *et al.* 1995).

- In situations of sustained, generalized HPV, pulmonary hypertension results. This pulmonary hypertension, induced primarily by chronic hypoxia, establishes with time and as a consequence secondary changes may occur in the pulmonary vasculature. These include muscle hypertrophy and intimal thickening.

- Many lung diseases not only cause hypoxia (inducing HPV and therefore pulmonary hypertension), but also destroy the vascular bed, contributing to increased vascular resistance and raised pulmonary artery pressures. A common example of this 'double' mechanism is severe CAL.

- In patients with CAL, the correct use of oxygen therapy may delay the onset of pulmonary hypertension, or partially reverse existing hypertension; this will ultimately improve survival (Bernard *et al.* 1995) (c.f. oxygen therapy).

Related topics

ACBT +/− manual techniques (p. 71); CPAP (p. 76); GAP (p. 129); IPPB (p. 99); Mobilization (p. 113); Mechanical ventilation (p. 109); NIPPV (p. 118); Oxygen therapy (p. 122); Positioning to maximize ventilation–perfusion ratio (p. 136).

References and further reading

Barnes P.J. and Liu S.F. (1995) Regulation of pulmonary vascular tone. *Pharmacol Rev* **47**: 87–131.

Bernard G.R., Rinaldo J., Harris T. *et al.* (1985) Early predictors of ARDS reversal in patients with established ARDS. *Am Rev Resp Dis* **131**: A143 (abstract).

Fishman A.P. (1961) Respiratory gases in the regulation of the pulmonary circulation. *Physiol Rev* **41**: 214–280.

Michel C.C. and Milledge J.S. (1963) Respiratory regulation in man during acclimatisation to high altitude. *J Physiol* **168**: 631.

Severinghaus J.W. (1992) Respiratory control related to altitude and anaesthesia. In: *Anaesthesia and the Lung* (eds T.H. Stanley and R.J. Sperry). Dordrecht, Kluwer, p. 97.

Wagner P.D. and Rodriquez-Roisin R. (1991) Clinical advances in pulmonary gas exchange. *Am Rev Respir Dis* **143**: 883.

Ward M.P., Milledge J.S. and West J.B. (1989) In: *High Altitude Medicine and Physiology*. Chapman and Hall, London.

Weinberger S.E., Schwartzstein R.M. and Weiss W. (1989) Hypercapnia. *N Engl J Med* **321**: 1223.

West J.B. (1990) *Ventilation/Blood Flow and Gas Exchange*. 5th edition. Blackwell, Oxford.

West J.B. (1995) *Pulmonary Pathophysiology*. 5th edition. Williams and Wilkins, Baltimore.

IMPAIRED TRACHEOBRONCHIAL CLEARANCE

Description

The lungs are exposed to a constant barrage of environmental insults. Mucociliary clearance and normal breathing (2 phase flow) are the principal methods employed to clear the lungs of inhaled foreign particles and endogenous cell debris. The cough mechanism is essential when these primary mechanisms are dysfunctional or overwhelmed.

Key physiological principles

Mucociliary clearance

- The mucociliary system comprises the cilia, mucus and periciliary fluid.
- The cilia rest with the tips in direct contact with the mucus blanket. The cilia beat with a co-ordinated *effective* and *recovery* stroke, propelling the mucus away from the terminal bronchioles. The mucus is then swallowed or expectorated.
- Cilia appear to be continuously active, with a variety of mediators involved in the modulation of beat frequency.
- Mucus is a gel layer overlying the cilia. It has characteristics of both a liquid (viscosity) and a solid (elasticity).
- The 'solid' characteristic allows the cilia to perform the transport function efficiently and effectively. The 'liquid' characteristic allows diffusion of water and solutes (maintaining epithelial hydration), dilutes/traps inhaled foreign substances, and permits deployment of antibacterial defenses.
- Mucus also demonstrates thixotropy, i.e. at high stress (e.g. cough), mucus viscosity is low, whilst at low stress (e.g. gravity) mucus viscosity is high.
- Mucus is secreted by a number of cells throughout the tracheobronchial tree. It is probable that afferent impulses from sensory fibers in the airways cause reflex mucus production. Mucus-secreting cells are stimulated via sympathetic, parasympathetic and non-adrenergic non-cholinergic pathways.
- Sputum is pathological mucus containing products of inflammation.
- Periciliary fluid is assumed to be a low-viscosity fluid bathing the cilia. It is thought to govern the composition of mucus and be regulated by active ion transport systems in the alveoli.

2 phase flow

- Normal breathing or 2 phase flow, facilitates tracheobronchial clearance. During expiration, the airways are narrower resulting in faster airflow and increased shear stress. Both factors favor the movement of mucus towards the mouth. During inspiration (reduced shear stress) the increase in mucus viscosity resists movement with airflow down the tracheobronchial tree.

Cough

- The cough reflex may be elicited by stimulation of the larynx, trachea, carina, main bronchi and airways. The process involves a large inspiration, contraction of expiratory muscles against a closed glottis (increasing intrapulmonary pressure), and finally an explosive expiration through narrowed airways as the glottis re-opens. The cough reflex effectively sweeps irritants from the large airways towards the mouth.

- It remains unclear as to which airway generation the cough may effectively clear.

Clinical relevance

- Impaired mucociliary clearance has been demonstrated in cystic fibrosis, chronic bronchitis, asthma, primary ciliary dyskinesia, common cold, acute lung infections, inhalation injury, bronchiectasis and during general anesthesia.
- Physiological factors known to adversely affect mucociliary clearance include increasing age and sleep. Conversely, exercise enhances mucociliary clearance.
- Smoking has been associated with increased numbers of abnormal cilia.
- Although ciliary dysfunction may occur as a result of structural abnormalities, ciliary absence or discordant beating, mucus abnormality may also be implicated. The inflammatory products present in pathological mucus may cause overwhelming mucus hypersecretion, or alter mucus rheology rendering it difficult to transport (c.f. inflammation).
- Bacterial and viral infection also cause reduced ciliary beat frequency, cell damage, altered ion transport and increased mucus production. A destructive, perpetual cycle may be established (c.f. infection).
- Poorly transported mucus is characterized by a lower salt concentration compared to normal mucus. Experimentally, addition of hypertonic saline solution rapidly improves mucociliary clearance. This has been exploited in the use of nebulized hypertonic saline solution for sputum induction. Isotonic saline and water have not been shown to accelerate tracheobronchial clearance *in vivo* (c.f. humidification).
- Pharmacological agents proposed to enhance tracheobronchial clearance include mucolytics (e.g. N-acetylcysteine, dornase alfa), and mucokinetics (e.g. hypertonic saline, β-agonists and aminophylline).
- The clinician must recognize when tracheobronchial clearance is impaired, facilitating secretion removal in other ways (c.f. ACBT, AD, Flutter, GAP, IPPB, MHI, manual techniques, mobilization, PEP, suction).
- Forced expiratory maneuvers and exercise are known to favor mucus expulsion. This is in part attributable to mucus thixotropy, i.e. the increased shear stress during the expiratory phase reduces the viscosity of mucus, thus facilitating its movement with airflow (c.f. ACBT).
- An individual's ability to cough may be impaired by recurrent laryngeal nerve palsy, tracheal intubation, pain, reduced consciousness or neuromuscular disease. In a patient with an impaired cough, a decline in the efficiency of mucociliary clearance may cause marked decompensation.
- In individuals with a reduced level of consciousness, a cough may be elicited by external tracheal stimulation above the sternal notch. In intubated patients, a cough may be elicited by instillation of normal saline and/or suction (c.f. tracheal suction). In patients with excessive mucus, a change in posture will often stimulate a cough (c.f. GAP, mobilization).

- Coughing is associated with large pressure changes in the thorax, arterial blood and cerebrospinal fluid. These changes may be more significant in compromised patients, e.g. reactive bronchospasm, small airway closure, syncope, raised intracranial pressure.

Related topics

ACBT+/– manual techniques (p. 71); Humidification (p. 94); GAP (p. 129); IPPB (p. 99); Mobilization (p. 113); Tracheal suction (p. 145); Tracheostomy management (p. 148).

References and further reading

Houtmeyers E., Gosselink R., Gayan-Ramirez G. and Decramer M. (1999) Regulation of mucociliary clearance in health and disease. *Euro Respir J* 13: 1177–1188.

Houtmeyers E., Gosselink R., Gayan-Ramirez G. and Decramer M. (1999) Effects of drugs on mucus clearance. *Euro Respir J* 14: 452–467.

Van der Schans C.P., Postma D.S., Koeter G.H. and Rubin B.K. (1999) Physiotherapy and bronchial mucus transport. *Euro Respir J* 13: 1477–1486.

INFECTION AND INFLAMMATION 1 – INFECTION

Description

Infection occurs when micro-organisms invade and multiply in normally sterile body tissue causing local cellular injury and an overt inflammatory response. Bacteremia is defined by the presence of viable bacteria in the blood.

Key physiological principles

- Resistance to infection is provided by physical (e.g. the GI tract), cellular (e.g. WBC – neutrophils, macrophages), inflammatory (e.g. cytokines, mediators) and humoral (e.g. antibody production) host defenses.
- A breakdown in any one of these components may lead to established infection.
- Deficiency in the barrier to infection may be temporary and will resolve with treatment/resolution of the underlying pathology (e.g. presence of an indwelling line, administration of immunosuppressant therapy).
- Long-term or permanent break down of the barrier to infection may be associated with HIV or malignancy, etc.

Clinical relevance

- The World Health Organization report 1998 (cited by Bion *et al.* 2001) identifies infection as the second commonest cause of death after cardiovascular disease. Infection may be community or hospital acquired.
- Nosocomial or hospital-acquired infections are prevalent. The majority are attributable to urinary tract, lower respiratory tract or surgical wound infection. Contributory factors include use of invasive lines/tubes/catheters, presence of pathogenic organisms within the hospital, multiresistant micro-organisms and 'immunodeficient' states.
- Respiratory tract infection is a general term covering a wide spectrum of infective conditions including pneumonia.
- Pneumonia is a complex pathological process that includes accumulation of inflammatory cells and exudate in the normally sterile lung parenchyma, in response to invasion and multiplication of micro-organisms. It may be discrete (lobar) or generalized (bronchopneumonia).
- Pneumonia may be nonproductive or productive of sputum. Physiotherapy treatment should be based on a thorough assessment of the presenting clinical signs and symptoms (c.f. ACBT, IPPB, GAP, manual techniques).
- Isolation of the infecting organism is beneficial in order to select the appropriate antibiotic/antiviral/antifungal.
- The spectrum of organisms is diverse for community-acquired pneumonia, hospital-acquired pneumonia and ventilator-associated pneumonia. Isolation of a causative organism is not always possible or reliable, therefore, empirical

antibiotic administration is often employed to cover likely or multiple organisms.

- During the last 20 years, Gram-positive cocci have developed marked antibiotic resistance (e.g. MRSA). Control measures should be implemented such as policies to curtail inappropriate antibiotic prescription, and isolation of colonized patients.
- All health care staff must be committed to infection control. Local guidelines regarding hygiene must be observed (c.f. tracheal suction, tracheostomy management).

Related topics

Infection and inflammation 2: Inflammation (p. 51); Sepsis (p. 56).

References and further reading

Bion J.F., Elliott T.S.J. and Glen L. (2001) Infection on the intensive care unit: the scale of the problem. In: Galley H.F. (ed). *Critical Care Focus. Antibiotic Resistance and Infection Control.* BMJ Books, London.

Sommers C. (1998) Immunity and inflammation. In: Mattson-Porth C. (ed). *Pathophysiology – Concepts of Altered Health States.* Lippincott, Philadelphia, pp. 189–210.

INFECTION AND INFLAMMATION 2 – INFLAMMATION

Description

Inflammation describes the reaction associated with injury (e.g. infection, trauma, surgery, thermal, irritant, ischemia) in vascularized tissue. The extent of the inflammatory response may be highly variable between individuals for the same stimulus and is aimed at minimizing tissue damage. Inflammatory conditions may be acute or chronic, localized or systemic.

This section will consider localized inflammation. Systemic inflammatory response syndrome (SIRS) is considered elsewhere.

Key physiological principles

- The five cardinal signs of inflammation are: erythema, edema, heat, pain and loss of function. These changes may be local and systemic.
- A cocktail of chemicals, including histamine, plasma proteases (kinins), prostaglandins, leukotrienes, and platelet-activating factor mediate the inflammatory response.
- Acute inflammation produces several distinct responses:
  - vascular responses: hyperemia and increased tissue permeability (resulting in inflammatory exudate);
  - cellular responses: marked white blood cell migration resulting in phagocytosis (engulfment and degradation of infective organisms and cell debris);
  - systemic responses: including fever, lethargy, increased erythrocyte sedimentation rate, increased white cell count, increased synthesis of C-reactive protein (c.f. SIRS).
- Chronic inflammation occurs when host defenses do not rapidly control a stimulus and may self-perpetuate indefinitely.
- Chronic inflammation may be initiated by persistent irritants (e.g. asbestos), infective organisms, injured tissue or immunological mechanisms.
- The responses to chronic inflammation are somewhat different, most notably the proliferation of fibroblasts resulting in tissue remodeling and scarring.

Clinical relevance

- Asthma is a chronic inflammatory disease of the airways associated with widespread and variable airflow limitation that may be partially or totally relieved by treatment/spontaneously. Uncontrolled, the chronic inflammatory process may result in functional and structural alterations, producing a hyper-responsive state (c.f. airflow limitation).
- Mortality associated with asthma is paralleled by the increasing prevalence of the disease worldwide.

- A modern approach to the management of asthma places a greater emphasis on disease modification than symptom modification. Prophylaxis and treatment/control of inflammation have become the new focus.
- It is recognized that health professionals need to develop a partnership of care with asthmatic patients, promoting education and principles of self-management. Improvements in self-management have been associated with a reduction in 'incidents' (e.g. consultations, exacerbations, need for steroids) and improved quality of life.
- Asthma, and other chronic inflammatory lung diseases (e.g. CAL, cystic fibrosis, bronchiectasis) are characteristically associated with impaired gas exchange and increased work of breathing.
- Chronic inflammation is also associated with interstitial lung disease, e.g. fibrosing alveolitis, sarcoidosis, Langerhan's hystiocytosis or organizing pneumonia. Ongoing infection leads to progressive lung fibrosis and a restrictive defect. Treatment invariably involves immunosuppression therapy (e.g. steroids, cyclophosphamide, methotrexate), which may predispose the patient to further infection (c.f. infection).
- Inflammation of the pleura (pleuritis) may be associated with pain and an altered pattern of breathing. Pleuritis may be acute, e.g. PE, infection/pneumonia or chronic, e.g. malignancy. Pleuritis may be associated with pleural effusion, and lead to altered chest wall dynamics (c.f. chest wall dysfunction/deformity).
- Surgical intervention or chest trauma will produce local inflammation and pain. This may be associated with chest wall dysfunction and a subsequent altered pattern of breathing, resulting in hypoventilation, atelectasis, sputum retention and an impaired cough (c.f. chest wall dysfunction/deformity, reduced lung volumes, impaired tracheobronchial clearance).
- Smoke inhalation injury is associated with mucosal inflammation.
- Upper airway inflammation, e.g. epiglottitis, acute laryngeal edema or pharyngeal infection may lead to upper airway obstruction and stridor. This condition may be misdiagnosed as asthma but is potentially life threatening and should be reported to medical staff immediately.
- An appreciation of the inflammatory process is also essential for directing effective pain management. The physiotherapist should be familiar with pharmacological and physiotherapeutic modalities which may modify aspects of the inflammatory response (c.f. pain, physiotherapy management of pain).

Related topics

References and further reading

BTS guidelines on asthma management: 1995 review and position statement (1997). *Thorax* 52 (Suppl).

Sears M.R. (2000) Consequences of long-term inflammation. The natural history of asthma. *Clin Chest Med* 21(2): 315–329.

Sommers C. (1998) Immunity and inflammation. In: Mattson-Porth C. (ed) *Pathophysiology – Concepts of Altered Health States*. Lippincott, Philadelphia, pp. 189–210.

INFECTION AND INFLAMMATION 3 – SEPSIS AND SYSTEMIC INFLAMMATORY RESPONSE SYNDROME (SIRS)

Description

Sepsis is the systemic inflammatory response to infection. Epidemiological studies have revealed that tissue injury secondary to activation of the inflammatory system may also occur with noninfectious disorders, e.g. acute pancreatitis and ischemia–reperfusion. The term systemic inflammatory response syndrome (SIRS) is used to refer to the consequences of a deregulated host inflammatory response when infection is not present. Therefore, in sepsis, the clinical signs of SIRS are present, together with definitive evidence of infection.

SIRS is a widespread inflammatory response to a variety of severe clinical insults. This syndrome is clinically recognized by the presence of two or more of the following:

- temperature >38°C or <36°C;
- heart rate >90 beats/min;
- respiratory rate >20 breaths/min or $PaCO_2$ <32 mmHg;
- WBC >12 000 cells/mm^3, <4000 cells/mm^3, or >10% immature (band) forms. (American College of Chest Physicians/Society of Critical Care Medicine 1992)

Key physiological principles

- Sepsis is a clinical syndrome, which complicates severe infection. It is characterized by systemic inflammation and widespread tissue injury.
- Sepsis is a syndrome in which tissues at a distance from the original insult show the main signs of inflammation, e.g. vasodilation, increased microvascular permeability, and leukocyte accumulation.
- Inflammation is a normal and essential host response, therefore, it is currently believed that the onset and progression of sepsis center upon a 'dysregulation' of the normal response, which produces a massive and uncontrolled release of proinflammatory mediators creating a chain of events that leads to widespread tissue injury.
- Sepsis is characterized by marked multisystem physiological derangements.
- Sepsis is considered severe when it is associated with organ dysfunction, hypoperfusion, or hypotension. The manifestations of hypoperfusion may include, but are not limited to, lactic acidosis, oliguria, or an acute alteration in mental status.
- In sepsis, abnormalities in coagulation and fibrinolysis are observed, including activation of the complement and coagulation systems. This produces a hypercoaguable state.
- Deposition of fibrin in the microvasculature is linked to development of multiple organ failure (MOF) and disseminated intravascular coagulation (DIC). These factors contribute to the poor prognosis associated with sepsis.
- MOF describes the presence of organ dysfunction in an acutely ill patient, such that homeostasis cannot be maintained without intervention.

- Septic shock is sepsis with hypotension (despite adequate fluid resuscitation), combined with hypoperfusion. Patients who are on inotropic or vasopressor agents may not be hypotensive at the time that perfusion abnormalities are measured.

Clinical relevance

- Sepsis affects up to 25% of all patients in an intensive care unit. Associated mortality with sepsis may exceed 50%, particularly in patients who develop organ failure and septic shock.
- Host-defense depression caused by co-morbidities (neoplasms, renal or hepatic failure, AIDS) is common in septic patients.
- The severity of sepsis can be related to several clinical characteristics including an abnormal host response to infection, the site and type of infection, the timing and type of antimicrobial therapy, and the development of shock.
- Risk factors for mortality from sepsis include age above 40 years and co-morbid conditions at the time of diagnosis of sepsis, e.g. AIDS, hepatic failure, cirrhosis, hematological malignancies, metastatic cancer, or immune suppression (Knaus *et al.* 1992).
- The most common manifestations of severe organ dysfunction are the acute respiratory distress syndrome, acute renal failure, and disseminated intra-vascular coagulation. Survival is reduced in patients with these complications.
- Many patients will require mechanical ventilation (c.f. mechanical ventilation).
- To date, there is no specific, beneficial treatment for sepsis, although future possibilities may involve replenishment of anticoagulant factors and proteins. Supportive care, particularly early provision of nutrition and prevention/treatment of nosocomial infections, is likely to improve outcome.
- The septic patient may be hemodynamically unstable. A clear indication must be present to warrant physiotherapy intervention. Increased inotropic support may be necessary to insure that an adequate blood pressure is maintained during treatment (c.f. manual hyperinflation).
- Careful positioning and passive movements (within the available range) are essential to maintain muscle and soft tissue length (c.f. mobilization, thoracic mobilization).

Related topics

Infection and inflammation 1: Infection (p. 51); Infection and inflammation 2: Inflammation (p. 53); Mechanical ventilation (p. 109).

References and further reading

American College of Chest Physicians/Society of Critical Care Medicine. (1992) Consensus Conference: Definitions for sepsis and organ failure and guidelines for the use of innovative therapies in sepsis. *Crit Care Med* 20: 864.
Knaus W.A., Sun X., Nystrom P.O. *et al.* (1992). Evaluation of definitions for sepsis. *Chest* **101**: 1656.

PAIN

Description

An unpleasant sensory and emotional experience associated with actual or potential tissue damage.

Key physiological principles

- Pain perception and modulation involves a complex series of events involving peripheral, spinal segmental, supraspinal and cortical levels (Walsh 1991).
- Pain can be described as being physiological or pathological.
- Physiological pain is the normal response to potentially damaging noxious stimuli. Activation of the nociceptors produces a localized, transient warning sign and protective withdrawal response. The amplitude of the response is proportional to the size of the stimulus.
- Pathological pain occurs secondary to nerve or tissue damage. It is characterized by disruption of the normal sensory mechanisms, so that pain occurs in the absence of a clear stimulus, e.g. allodynia (pain sensation in response to innocuous stimuli), hyperalgesia (amplified response to noxious stimuli) and hyperpathia (prolonged and exaggerated post-stimulus sensation).
- In the acute stages, pathological pain is a protective mechanism, allowing recuperation and repair. In chronic situations however, its function is unclear.
- Pathological pain is the result of nociceptive sensitization secondary to changes in the primary afferents (peripheral sensitization), or within the dorsal horn (central sensitization).
- In peripheral sensitization, products generated by tissue injury and neural factors cause sensitization of nociceptors and awakening of silent nociceptors. Activation of nociceptors may then occur spontaneously or with low-intensity stimuli.
- In central sensitization, a complex series of changes occur within the dorsal horn neurones (referred to as 'wind up') following nociceptor activity. This augments the response and causes it to outlast the duration of the stimulus, e.g. phantom limb pain.
- Visceral pain is deep and poorly localized. The nature of the stimulus may be distention, ischemia, inflammation or algesic chemicals.
- Referred pain (localization of pain in a distant structure) is located in areas/tissues innervated by the same spinal nerve as the affected viscous.
- Common examples of referred pain include arm, neck or jaw pain (cardiac) and shoulder tip pain (diaphragmatic or pleural).

Clinical relevance

- Effective physiotherapy is dependent upon adequate analgesia.
- Liaison with the multiprofessional team and the pain services will assure optimal pain management.

- Accurate and regular assessment of pain is a fundamental part of its management. Tools include visual analog scales or verbal descriptions. Signs associated with pain may include increased heart/respiratory rate, increased blood pressure, reluctance to move, etc.

Pharmacological management of pain

- Non-steroidal anti-inflammatory drugs (NSAIDS): Block the synthesis of prostaglandins therefore counter an inflammatory response at tissue level. May be associated with gastric irritation, bronchospasm, and impairment of renal function/clotting.
- Paracetamol: A weak inhibitor of prostaglandin synthesis. Is associated with liver damage in overdose.
- Opioids: Modulate pain sensation via action within the central nervous system. Effective in moderate to severe pain, particularly visceral. Can be administered in a variety of ways e.g. orally, intramuscularly, intravenously, subcutaneously or as a constituent of epidural anesthesia/analgesia. May be associated with nausea and vomiting, drowsiness and respiratory depression. Tramadol has been shown to produce less respiratory depression and drowsiness. Opioids may be delivered via a patient-controlled analgesia system (PCAS) where the patient self-administers a preset dose via a simple handset system. A lockout interval prevents overdose.
- Psychotropic drugs: May be of value with chronic pain, e.g. tricyclic antidepressants and anticonvulsants.
- Inhalant analgesia: Anesthetic gas administered in quantities that produce analgesia but not loss of consciousness. Useful in the management of temporary pain.
- Combination compounds: e.g. opioid and paracetamol.
- Local anesthetic agents: May be administered via epidural (frequently in conjunction with small amounts of opioids), or regionally (e.g. intercostal nerve blocks). Epidural analgesia is associated with a reduction in postoperative length of stay. Sensorimotor function and cardiovascular stability should always be assessed prior to and during mobilization of a patient with an epidural.
- Multimodal therapy is likely to be most effective in managing pain.
- The concept of central sensitization has important implications for pain management and development of new analgesics. Ideally, the establishment of central sensitization should be prevented. However, once established, it should be recognized that therapies directed purely at preventing nociceptive activation in the periphery will be inadequate.

Related topics

Pain management (p. 126); Thoracic mobilization (p. 143).

References and further reading

McQuay H. and Moore A. (1998) *An Evidence-based Resource for Pain Relief.* Oxford University Press, Oxford.

Wall P.D. and Melzack R. (eds) (1994) *Textbook of Pain*, 3rd edition. Churchill Livingstone, Edinburgh.

Walsh D. (1991) Nociceptive Pathways – Relevance to The Physiotherapist. *Physiotherapy* 77(5): 317–321.

REDUCED LUNG VOLUME

Description

Reduction in lung volume is frequently multifactorial, and may be acute or chronic. This section will consider reduced lung volume with reference to:

- Vital capacity (VC): the volume of gas inhaled following a maximal exhalation.
- Tidal volume (V_T): the volume of gas inhaled during quiet 'tidal' breathing.
- Functional residual capacity (FRC): the remaining lung volume after quiet expiration.
- Closing capacity (CC): the lung volume at which dependent airways start to close.

Key physiological principles

The consequences of a reduction in lung volume are:

- Atelectasis in dependent lung – tidal breathing (and therefore FRC) occurs within CC range causing small airway closure.
- Perfusion of inadequately ventilated lung produces hypoxemia (c.f. impaired gaseous exchange).
- Increased airflow resistance due to reduced airway caliber increases work of breathing and predisposes to further airway collapse during forced expiratory maneuvers (c.f. airflow limitation).
- Reduced compliance – compliance falls with a reduction in lung volume (reflecting the curvilinearity of the pressure–volume curve), increasing work of breathing (c.f. altered respiratory compliance).
- Reduced efficacy cough secondary to reduction in VC.
- The extent of the impairment produced will depend upon the patient's co-morbidity and ability to compensate, e.g. an inability to increase respiratory rate to maintain an adequate minute volume may lead to respiratory failure (c.f. respiratory failure).

Clinical relevance

Causes of reduced lung volume include:

- Atelectasis, e.g. hypoventilation, pain, post-anesthetic, surfactant disturbance, mucus plugging, infection.
- Pain (c.f. pain, pain management).
- Compression, e.g. pleural effusions, ascites, obesity, pneumothorax, cardiomegaly.
- Reduced respiratory compliance, e.g. fibrotic lung disease, pneumonia, kyphoscoliosis (c.f. altered respiratory compliance).
- Respiratory muscle dysfunction, e.g. fatigue or weakness (c.f. respiratory muscle dysfunction).

- Posture, e.g. supine, slumped sitting (c.f. positioning to increase lung volume).
- Prophylactic preservation of lung volume should be considered in 'at-risk' groups, e.g. early mobilization for postoperative patients.
- In order to be able to maintain adequate spontaneous ventilation a VC >1 liter is required. Any patient with a significantly reduced VC should be assessed for ventilatory support (c.f. NIPPV, mechanical ventilation).
- Methods to increase V_T include controlled exercise, lower thoracic expansion exercises, selected neurophysiological facilitation techniques, MHI and IPPB.
- Areas with low lung volume are less compliant as they fall on the lower, flatter portion of the pressure–volume curve (c.f. altered respiratory compliance). Consequently it is important to insure that modalities such as lower thoracic expansion exercises and IPPB do not merely overinflate the more compliant regions. This is achieved by selecting appropriate positioning, insuring adequate relaxation, the use of breathing control and where possible slower inspiratory flow rates.
- Methods to increase FRC include controlled exercise, positioning, and CPAP/Bi-level positive airways pressure.
- Increasing tidal volume reduces resistance to airflow in collateral channels of ventilation and enhances the effect of interdependence (the expanding forces exerted between adjacent alveoli). Both these mechanisms may facilitate the re-expansion of alveoli at the point of collapse (c.f. IPPB).
- Lung volume may be reduced surgically in patients with severe emphysematous or bullous disease. This procedure aims to optimize lung mechanics by improving hyperinflated lung.

Related topics

CPAP (p. 76); Glossopharyngeal breathing (p. 92); IPPB (p. 99); Manual hyperinflation (p. 102); Mobilization (p. 113); NIPPV (p. 118); NPF (p. 115); Positioning to increase lung volume (p. 133).

References and further reading

Bancalari E. and Clausen J. (1998) Pathophysiology of changes in absolute lung volumes. *Eur Respir J* 12(1): 248–258.

Johnson N.T. and Pierson D.J. (1986). The spectrum of pulmonary atelectasis: pathophysiology, diagnosis and therapy. *Respir Care* 31(11): 1107–1120.

RESPIRATORY FAILURE

Description

Respiratory failure is defined as the inability to maintain the partial pressures in arterial blood of carbon dioxide (P_aCO_2) and oxygen (P_aO_2) within normal physiological limits.

Key physiological principles

Respiratory failure may occur as a result of:

- Failure of gas exchange due to lung disease ('Type 1' or 'hypoxemic' failure).
- Failure of the respiratory pump: chest wall, respiratory muscles, and/or central/peripheral neural components ('Type 2' or 'ventilatory' failure).
- Failure of either the gas exchange or respiratory pump component produces distinct pathophysiological features (c.f. impaired gaseous exchange, respiratory muscle dysfunction). However the two are frequently interlinked, and the presence of one invariably leads to the development or exacerbation of the other.
- Type 1 respiratory failure is characterized by hypoxemia with normo/hypocapnia. The underlying cause is a disturbance in ventilation–perfusion relationships within the lung.
- Patchy distribution of lung disease results in areas with reduced ventilation relative to perfusion. This produces a fall in P_aO_2 and rise in P_aCO_2. However, the rise in P_aCO_2 in these conditions is inconsequential as the arteriovenous difference is small. Eventually the P_aCO_2 may fall below normal levels, as the reduction in P_aO_2 stimulates the respiratory center to increase alveolar ventilation.
- In this situation increased ventilation is not sufficient to restore P_aO_2 to normal levels. This is due to the sigmoid shape of the oxygen dissociation curve. The increase in alveolar ventilation occurs mainly in the normally ventilated lung, where the oxygen content is already high. Oxygen content cannot be increased sufficiently to compensate for the diseased areas.
- Type 2 respiratory failure is characterized by hypercapnia secondary to alveolar hypoventilation.
- Alveolar hypoventilation results from disturbance of the respiratory pump, an unfavorable change in load, capacity, or central drive that cannot be compensated for by the patient.
- It is not clear whether the reduction in central drive represents primary failure or a self-preservation mechanism designed to prevent pushing the respiratory pump to total failure (c.f. respiratory muscle dysfunction).
- Sleep is normally associated with alterations in central drive and muscle tone. In vulnerable individuals, i.e. those with a precarious balance between central drive, capacity and load, sleep may lead to nocturnal hypoventilation and eventually diurnal respiratory failure (c.f. control of breathing).

Clinical relevance

Conditions predisposing to Type 1 failure include:

- pneumonia;
- pulmonary edema;
- pulmonary embolism;
- asthma;
- fibrosing alveolitis.

Conditions predisposing to Type 2 failure include:

- head injury;
- opiate overdose;
- cervical cord lesions;
- polio;
- Guillain–Barré syndrome;
- muscular dystrophy;
- myasthenia gravis;
- thoracic injury/deformity;
- CAL;
- cystic fibrosis.

- Respiratory failure may be an acute event, e.g. pulmonary embolus, acute on chronic, e.g. acute infective exacerbation of chronic airflow limitation, or chronic manifestation, e.g. neuromuscular disorders.
- Appropriate management is dependent upon identification and where possible, reversal of the underlying pathophysiological factors which have precipitated the respiratory failure. These may include reversal of pulmonary edema, drainage of a pleural effusion, appropriate treatment of infection, stabilization of the chest wall, reversal of sedation, removal of secretions, administration of analgesia, reversal of atelectasis, protection of the airway, treatment of bronchospasm, etc.
- First-line treatment is to relieve hypoxemia, where possible, via oxygen therapy, however, caution must be exercised in the presence of chronic CO_2 retention (c.f. oxygen therapy).
- Ventilatory assistance may be applied invasively or noninvasively. Noninvasive ventilation may be continuous, periodic or nocturnal.
- Criteria for considering ventilatory assistance include: respiratory rate >30/min, pH <7.2 kPa for intubation and 7.25–7.3 for NIPPV, exhaustion and/or confusion (c.f. mechanical ventilation, NIPPV).
- Patients with hypoperfusion states, e.g. cardiogenic, hypovolemic or septic shock frequently present with tachypnea and an abnormal respiratory pattern, in the absence of pulmonary problems. In these situations, mechanical ventilation stabilizes gas exchange and reduces the 'steal' of limited cardiac output by working respiratory muscles.

Related topics

CPAP (p. 76); IPPB (p. 99); Mechanical ventilation (p. 107); NIPPV (p. 118).

References and further reading

DeAnda G.F. and Lachmann B. (2001) Treatment and prevention of acute respiratory failure: physiological basis. *Arch Med Res* **32**(2): 91–101.

Gribbin H.R. (1993) Management of respiratory failure. *Br J Hosp Med* **49**(7): 461–477.

Hedenstierna G. and Neumann P. (1999) Gas exchange in acute respiratory failure. *Minerva Anesthesiol* **65**(6): 383–387.

Simonds A.K. (1996) Pathophysiology of ventilatory failure. In: Simonds A (ed). *Non-invasive Respiratory Support*. Chapman and Hall, London.

RESPIRATORY MUSCLE DYSFUNCTION

Description

The respiratory muscles, chest wall and the central nervous system form the 'respiratory pump' responsible for ventilating the lungs. The respiratory muscles include the diaphragm, intercostal, abdominal and accessory (neck and trunk) muscles. Dysfunction may be a result of fatigue and/or weakness.

- Fatigue: an exertion-induced reduction in the capacity to generate force that may be reversed by rest.
- Weakness: a reduction in the capacity of rested muscle to generate force. May predispose to fatigue.

Key physiological principles

- Under normal conditions, the inspiratory muscles generate sufficient force to overcome the elastic loads of the lungs and chest wall, and resistive loads of the airways and tissues. They possess the ability to maintain a reasonable load over time, as well as adjusting the minute volume to insure adequate gas exchange under various conditions.
- Respiratory muscle dysfunction is multifactorial and common in a wide range of conditions. Dysfunction is dependent upon a synergistic interplay between energy supply/demand, load and system competence, for example:
  - Reduced energy supply: e.g. hypoxemia, poor nutrition, reduced blood flow, impaired ability to extract nutrients, accumulation of breakdown products (c.f. impaired gaseous exchange).
  - Increased energy demand: muscles at a mechanical disadvantage because of altered length–tension relationship, e.g. hyperinflation or an unstable chest wall, persistent activity during expiration, e.g. severe asthma, elevated respiratory rate, excessive accessory muscle use (c.f. reduced lung volumes, airflow limitation, chest wall deformity/disruption).
  - Excessive load: e.g. increased airflow resistance or reduced respiratory compliance (c.f. altered respiratory compliance).
  - Reduced system competence: e.g. impaired central drive, abnormal impulse propagation or failure/weakness of the contractile apparatus (c.f. control of breathing).
- The majority of muscular work is performed during inspiration. Consequently the inspiratory muscles are those at greatest risk of developing fatigue.

Clinical relevance

- The consequences of respiratory muscle dysfunction range from mild dyspnea and exercise limitation to overt ventilatory failure. The clinical signs will vary accordingly.

- Clinical signs and symptoms indicative of acute and chronic dysfunction include:
  - Tachypnea (which may progress to bradypnea as central drive is reduced to prevent driving the muscles to failure/destruction) and dyspnea.
  - Paradoxical breathing. Paradoxical movement of the chest wall and/or abdomen during inspiration, e.g. diaphragmatic weakness: the abdomen moves in on inspiration as the weakened diaphragm is pulled up by transmission of the negative intrapleural pressure.
  - Respiratory alternans (phasic alterations between abdominal and thoracic breathing).
  - Impaired thoracic expansion and cough.
  - Accessory muscle use to supplement fatiguing respiratory muscles.
  - Symptoms of sleep-disordered breathing.
- Symptoms may be aggravated by position, e.g. the supine position in diaphragmatic weakness/fatigue.
- Further assessment may be undertaken via lung function testing, e.g. vital capacity, maximal inspiratory pressure.
- High spinal injuries are associated with marked respiratory muscle dysfunction. Lesions above C4 leave only accessory muscles and therefore necessitate ventilatory support. Lesions below C4 cause paralysis of the intercostal and abdominal muscles. For these patients respiratory paradox involves inward movement of the chest wall and outward bulging of the abdomen during inspiration. Additionally, the supine position may be favored by this group as the weight of the abdominal contents pushes the diaphragm to a higher resting level, giving it a mechanical advantage which is lost in the upright position. Abdominal muscle paralysis reduces active expiratory maneuvers and therefore external compression may be required.
- In all cases of respiratory muscle dysfunction, therapy should be directed not only at supporting/maintaining ventilation, but where possible addressing causes of dysfunction, e.g. relieving obstruction/hypoxemia, treating infection, inspiratory muscle training, etc. Prevention of further complications is also essential, e.g. secretion retention (c.f. ACBT, GAP, IPPB).
- Resting the respiratory muscles may be of benefit, e.g. mechanical ventilation, NIPPV.
- In chronic conditions, exercise training may be considered to prevent deconditioning as well as maximizing potential.

Related topics

Glossopharyngeal breathing (p. 92); IPPB (p. 99); Mechanical ventilation (p. 109); NIPPV (p. 118).

References and further reading

Mador M.J. (1991) Respiratory muscle fatigue and breathing pattern. *Chest* **100**: 1430–1435.

Moxham J. (1990) Respiratory muscle fatigue. *Br J Anaes* **65**: 43–53.

Polkey M.I. and Moxham J. (2001) Clinical aspects of respiratory muscle dysfunction in the critically ill. *Chest* **119**(3): 926–939.

Vassilakopoulos T., Zakynthinos S., Roussos C. *et al.* (1995) Respiratory muscle fatigue. *Intensive Care* **Autumn**: 85–95.

Section 3

PHYSIOTHERAPY TECHNIQUES AND ADJUNCTS

ACTIVE CYCLE OF BREATHING TECHNIQUES (ACBT)

Description

ACBT are a specific set of breathing exercises designed to remove excess bronchial secretions. The three key phases are: (1) breathing control (relaxation); (2) lower thoracic expansion exercises (active secretion mobilization); and (3) forced expiration technique (FET), (active secretion clearance).

Key physiological principles

- Effective ACBT requires appropriate positioning to optimize inspiratory muscle efficiency, match ventilation/perfusion and reduce unnecessary muscular activity. The position will be specific to each individual patient (c.f. Positioning to relieve breathlessness, positioning to maximize ventilation/perfusion ratio, positioning to improve lung volume).
- Breathing control is normal tidal breathing, incorporated to promote relaxation and prevent hyperventilation, and may assist the patient to tolerate the sensation of dyspnea. Consequently, treatment should commence with breathing control.
- Lower thoracic expansion exercises aim to actively increase lung volume above tidal volume. This results in:
  - reduced resistance to airflow via the collateral ventilation system;
  - enhanced interdependence (the expanding forces exerted by adjacent alveoli);
  - mobilization of secretions;
  - re-expansion of lung tissue at the point of sputum-related collapse (Tucker and Jenkins 1996).
- Mobilization of the thoracic cage, and increased strength, endurance and efficiency of the respiratory muscles have also been ascribed to the use of LTEE (Tucker and Jenkins 1996).
- The FET is a combination of 1–2 forced expiratory maneuvers ('huffs'), and breathing control. The huff produces dynamic compression of the airways proximal to the equal pressure point, i.e. the point at which the pressure inside the airway is equal to intrapleural pressure (West 1995). Repetition of this procedure facilitates movement of excess bronchial secretions towards the mouth.

Clinical relevance

Efficacy

- ACBT are effective and efficient in the removal of excess bronchial secretions (Pryor et al. 1979) producing an improvement in lung function in patients with cystic fibrosis (Webber et al. 1986).

- When the ACBT are used as described, there is no associated hypoxemia (Pryor *et al.* 1990) or increase in airway obstruction (Pryor *et al.* 1979)
- Secretion removal utilizing ACBT is not further enhanced by the additional use of PEP or flutter in the CF population (Hofmeyr *et al.* 1986, Pryor *et al.* 1994) (c.f. PEP, flutter).
- The divisions of the bronchial tree to which the ACBT have an effect has not been verified. However, it is generally believed that ACBT may be effective even in distal airways.

Mechanism of FET

- When a patient performs a forced expiratory maneuver from a lung volume greater than FRC, the equal pressure point is located in or above the lobar or segmental bronchi, thus mobilizing secretions from the larger more proximal airways (Macklem 1974).
- The use of a forced expiratory maneuver to a mid/low lung volume generates an equal pressure point further from the mouth, therefore mobilizing secretions from the smaller more distal airways (Pryor 1999).
- Oscillatory motion of the airway walls has been shown to occur in addition to dynamic compression during a forced expiratory maneuver, which may contribute to mobilization of secretions (Freitag *et al.* 1989).
- FET versus cough: Both effectively clear secretions, but FET requires less effort (Hasani *et al.* 1994). Furthermore, coughing is associated with greater compression and narrowing of the airways due to high mean transpulmonary pressure. This limits airflow and therefore may impede secretion clearance (Langlands 1967).
- The huff should never be a violently forced maneuver. The nature of the huff may be manipulated to address specific requirements, e.g. varying length and force of contraction to maximize peripheral secretion clearance or minimize airway closure. However, a violent or excessively prolonged huff may promote coughing and/or airway closure, whilst too short a huff will be ineffective.

Indications for use

- Clinically, these techniques are widely used in the management of any spontaneously breathing patient presenting with excess bronchial secretions (c.f. impaired tracheobronchial clearance).
- The component parts of the ACBT can be manipulated to meet individual patient requirements, e.g. longer periods of breathing control in the breathless patient or the addition of an inspiratory hold in a post-surgical patient.
- The FET is a useful adjunct to treatment in the surgical patient. Wound compression by the patient or physiotherapist and adequate analgesia are recommended to minimize potential discomfort.
- ACBT can be combined with other physiotherapeutic techniques to meet individual patients needs, e.g. GAP, manual techniques and exercise (c.f. GAP, manual techniques, exercise training).
- ACBT is an important component of patient self-management, therefore, regular reassessment of each patient's requirements is essential to maintain treatment adherence (Carr *et al.* 1996).

Related topics

Airflow limitation (p. 17); Control of breathing (p. 26); Effects of general anesthesia (p. 41); Impaired gaseous exchange (p. 44); Impaired tracheobronchial clearance (p. 48); Reduced lung volume (p. 61).

References and further reading

Carr L., Smith R., Pryor J. and Partridge C. (1996) CF patients views and beliefs about chest clearance and exercise. *Physiotherapy* **82**: 612–616

Freitag L., Bremme R. and Schroer M. (1989) High frequency oscillation for respiratory physiotherapy. *Br J Anaes* **63**: 44s–46s

Hasani A., Pavia D., Agnew J. and Clarke S. (1994) Regional lung clearance during cough and FET: Effects of flow and viscoelasticity. *Thorax* **49**: 557–561.

Hofmeyr J.L., Webber B.A. and Hodson M.E. (1986) Evaluation of PEP as an adjunct to chest physiotherapy in the treatment of cystic fibrosis. *Thorax* **41**: 951–954.

Langlands J. (1967) The dynamics of cough in health and in chronic bronchitis. *Thorax* **22**: 88–96

Macklem P. (1974) *Physiology of Cough.* Transactions of the American Broncho-Esophogological Association, pp. 150–157

Pryor J.A. (1999) Physiotherapy for airway clearance in adults. *Eur Respir J* **14**: 1418–1424.

Pryor J.A., Webber B., Hodson M. and Batten J. (1979) Evaluation of the FET as an adjunct to postural drainage in treatment of CF. *BMJ* **2**: 417–418.

Pryor J.A., Webber B. and Hodson M. (1990) Effect of chest physiotherapy on oxygen saturation in patients with CF. *Thorax* **45**: 77.

Pryor J.A., Webber B., Hodson M. and Warner J. (1994) The Flutter VRPI as an adjunct to chest physiotherapy in CF. *Respir Med* **88**: 677–681.

Tucker B. and Jenkins S. (1996) The effect of breathing exercises with body positioning on regional lung ventilation. *Aust J Physio* **42**(3): 219–227.

Webber B., Hofmeyr J., Morgan M. and Hodson M. (1986) Effects of postural drainage, incorporating the FET, on pulmonary function in CF. *Br J Dis Chest* **80**: 353–359.

West J. (1995) *Pulmonary Pathophysiology*, 5th edition. Williams & Wilkins, Baltimore.

AUTOGENIC DRAINAGE

Description

Autogenic drainage (AD) combines the technique of breathing control with breaths taken at various lung volumes. Airflow is maximized, in order to improve mucus clearance and ventilation. The three key phases are: (1) 'unstick' (breathing at low lung volume – active secretion mobilization); (2) 'collect' (breathing around tidal volume); and (3) 'evacuate' (breathing at high lung volume – active expectoration of secretions).

Key physiological principles

- The active part of this technique aims to achieve the greatest possible airflow through the bronchi. The augmented inspiratory volume employed during this 'unstick' phase is thought to mobilize secretions from distal lung units via compression of peripheral alveolar ducts (Kraemer *et al.* 1986).
- Controlled tidal breathing is then used to 'collect' mobilized secretions. During the 'collect' phase, breathing starts in the expiratory reserve volume and progresses sequentially to the inspiratory reserve volume. This is thought to mobilize secretions from both distal and proximal segments respectively (Kraemer *et al.* 1986).
- The exhalation, which follows, uses a high expiratory flow rate, essential to mobilize secretions (Schoni 1989). During this 'evacuation' phase, the velocity of airflow is controlled throughout allowing movement of secretions distal to the equal pressure points generated (Kraemer *et al.* 1986, Schoni 1989).

Clinical relevance

- Developed in Belgium by Jean Chevaillier in the late 1960s, and was brought to England in the late 1970s (Dab & Alexander 1979).
- German therapists (David 1991) later simplified the original Belgian approach in which the three phases are no longer split (Kieselmann 1995).

Efficacy

- AD is usually performed in the sitting position, which may potentially limit effective basal clearance.
- AD requires up to 20 hours tuition to learn the basic principles. Effective treatment requires twice daily sessions of up to 45 minutes duration (David 1991).
- The Belgian method is rarely performed effectively as patients find breathing at low to mid lung volumes uncomfortable to maintain (Schoni 1989).
- A long-term study involving patients with cystic fibrosis, compared AD to 'conventional physiotherapy' (GAP and percussion) (c.f. GAP, manual techniques). AD was found to be as effective as conventional treatment. In addition, the patients preferred AD as a treatment modality (Davidson *et al.* 1992).
- Miller *et al.* (1995), performed a comparative study of AD and ACBT/GAP.

They reported no difference in effectiveness between these two techniques, and subjects reported a preference for AD. However, it is noted that four subjects desaturated during treatment with ACBT/GAP. ACBT/GAP correctly performed, should not cause desaturation. This questions the accuracy of the techniques performed in this trial (c.f. ACBT).

- AD was found to be as effective as the ACBT in aiding secretion clearance and improving lung function in CAL patients (Savci *et al.* 2000).
- AD is both time consuming to teach and difficult to master, therefore, there may be no additional benefit in using AD as a treatment modality over the ACBT.

Indications for use
- Removal of excess bronchial secretions.

Contraindications
- AD is unsuitable for the treatment of children under 8 years of age due to the prolonged periods of concentration required.

Related topics

Impaired gaseous exchange (p. 44); Impaired tracheobronchial clearance (p. 48).

References and further reading

Dab I. and Alexander F. (1979) The mechanism of autogenic drainage studied with flow–volume curves. *Monograph Paediat* **10**: 50–53.

David A. (1991) Autogenic drainage – The German approach. In: Pryor JA (ed) *Respiratory Care*. Churchill Livingstone, Edinburgh, pp. 65–78.

Davidson A.G.F., Wong L.T.K., Pirie G.E. and McIlwaine P.M. (1992) Long term comparative trial of conventional percussion and drainage physiotherapy versus autogenic drainage in cystic fibrosis. *Paediatric Pulmonology* **8** (suppl): 298.

Kieselmann R. (1995) Modified AD. In: *Physiotherapy in the Treatment of Cystic Fibrosis*, 2nd edition. International Physiotherapy Group for Cystic Fibrosis (IPG/CF), pp. 13–14.

Kraemer R., Zumbuhl C., Rudeberg A., Lentze M.J. and Chevaillier J. (1986) Autogene Drainage bei Patienten mit zystischer Fibrose. *Padiatrische Praxis* **3**: 223–232.

Miller S., Hall D.O., Clayton C.B. and Nelson R. (1995) Chest physiotherapy in CF: a comparative study of autogenic drainage and the active cycle of breathing techniques with postural drainage. *Thorax* **50**(2): 165–169.

Savci S., Ince D.I. and Arikan H. (2000) A comparison of autogenic drainage and the active cycle of breathing techniques in patients with COPD. *J Cardiopulm Rehabil* **20**(1): 37–43.

Schoni M.H. (1989) Autogenic drainage: a modern approach to physiotherapy in cystic fibrosis. *J Royal Soc Med* **82** (suppl 16): 32–37.

CONTINUOUS POSITIVE AIRWAYS PRESSURE

Description

The application of supra-atmospheric pressure throughout the respiratory cycle in spontaneously breathing patients. The first clinical trials were described in 1936 (Poulton and Oxon 1936), when a vacuum cleaner was used to generate the gas flow!

Key physiological principles

- Continuous positive airways pressure (CPAP) is associated with an increase in FRC, leading to a reduced shunt fraction, improved lung compliance, improved arterial saturation and diminished work associated with breathing (Denehy and Berney 2001).
- The postulated mechanism underlying the increase in FRC is related to collateral channels of ventilation. It is suggested that the increase in lung volume during CPAP application reduces collateral flow resistance and therefore promotes collateral flow to obstructed lung regions (Andersen *et al.* 1979).

Clinical relevance

Efficacy

- CPAP has been shown to be effective in the treatment of acute (Type 1) respiratory failure, pulmonary contusion and flail chest, cardiogenic pulmonary edema, obstructive sleep apnea and atelectasis (postoperative or secondary to neurological disease/insult) (Denehy and Berney 2001, Simonds 1996) (c.f. respiratory failure, mechanical ventilation, reduced lung volumes).
- CPAP may also be effective in patients with an acute exacerbation of CAL, although NIPPV may be a more appropriate method of support if the P_aCO_2 is markedly elevated or climbing (Simonds 1996). Caution should be exercised when using CPAP in patients with hyperinflated lungs (c.f. airflow limitation).
- The use of prophylactic CPAP postoperatively has been investigated with conflicting results (Denehy and Berney 2001).
- The increase in FRC is proportional to the level of CPAP applied (Gherini *et al.* 1979) (c.f. reduced lung volumes).
- Recruitment of the channels of collateral ventilation during CPAP application may have a potential secretion clearing effect. Collateral ventilation may allow airflow behind secretions, thereby promoting airway clearance (Denehy and Berney 2001) (c.f. impaired tracheobronchial clearance).
- The efficacy of periodic CPAP remains unclear. The time course of changes in lung volume with application and removal of positive end expiratory pressure have been reported to be less than 1 minute (Katz *et al.* 1981), and many other factors are likely to contribute to the extent of treatment carry-over.
- The optimal treatment regime for the use of CPAP as a physiotherapy treatment has not been established (Denehy and Berney 2001).

Indications for use

- Conditions characterized by a reduction in FRC (with associated decline in respiratory function and gas exchange), where voluntary lung expansion techniques are not effective or appropriate (Denehy and Berney 2001).

Application

- CPAP can be applied via a facemask, nasal mask, mouthpiece, flange or ETT/tracheostomy tube.
- Nasal CPAP is much less effective if the patient mouth breathes. Loss of airway pressure results in unreliable levels of CPAP. In this situation a full facemask is indicated.
- An effective CPAP flow generator should be able to provide flow rates in excess of the patient's peak inspiratory flow (approximately 35–40 l/min).
- The CPAP flow generator allows the manipulation of FiO_2 in order to maintain adequate oxygenation (c.f. oxygen therapy).
- A positive end expiratory pressure (PEEP) valve between 2.5–20 cmH_2O is used to elevate end expiratory pressure. Appropriate selection of the PEEP level is based on patient size, pathology and response to treatment.
- For the purposes of physiotherapy ≥ 10 cmH_2O applied for 30 minutes (if tolerated), 1–2 hourly is recommended (Denehy and Berney 2001).
- A safety valve 5 cmH_2O above the selected PEEP should be incorporated into the circuit to allow an 'escape' route in case of obstruction.
- Humidification is essential for continuous CPAP in view of the high flow rates. Heated devices offer the most effective humidification (c.f. humidification).

Contraindications and cautions

- The absolute contraindication to CPAP is an undrained pneumothorax.
- The potential adverse effects associated with CPAP are cardiovascular instability secondary to increased intrathoracic pressure (particularly in the presence of hypovolemia), barotrauma (rare), hypoventilation and carbon dioxide retention.
- Mask CPAP may also be associated with nasal bridge sores, gastric distention and aspiration.
- Caution must be exercised and appropriate monitoring commenced when using mask CPAP in drowsy patients or those at risk of vomiting.
- Mask CPAP should only be undertaken with extreme caution in patients with unstable facial fractures or severe facial lacerations, laryngeal trauma, raised intracranial pressure, basal skull fractures, severe hyperinflated lung disease and recent esophageal or tracheal anastamoses.
- CPAP affects antidiuretic hormone (ADH) production, therefore urine output should be monitored in vulnerable patients.

Related topics

References and further reading

Andersen J., Ovist J. and Kann H. (1979) Recruiting collapsed lung through collateral channels with positive end expiratory pressure. *Scand J Respir Dis* **60**: 260–266.

Denehy L. and Berney S. (2001) The use of positive pressure devices by physiotherapists. *Eur Respir J* **17**: 821–829.

Gherini S., Peters R. and Virgilio R. (1979) Mechanical work of the lungs and work of breathing with positive end expiratory pressure and continuous positive airway pressure. *Chest* **76**: 251–256.

Katz J., Ozanne G., Zinn S. and Fairly B. (1981) Time course and mechanisms of lung volume increase with PEEP in acute pulmonary failure. *Anaesthesiology* **54**: 9–16.

Poulton E. and Oxon D. (1936) Left sided heart failure with pulmonary oedema: Its treatment with the 'pulmonary plus pressure machine'. *Lancet* **231**: 981–983.

Simonds A.K. (1996) *Non-invasive Respiratory Support*. Chapman and Hall Medical, London.

EXERCISE TRAINING 1

Description

Exercise is any and all activity involving generation of force by the activated muscles, which results in disruption of a homeostatic state (American College of Sports Medicine, cited by McArdle *et al.* 1996). Exercise performance can be improved with training and is an example of biological long-term adaptation to increased chronic stress (Fletcher *et al.* 1996). The principal objective of training is to facilitate adaptations that improve performance in specific tasks.

Key physiological principles

- Training is exercise specific. Strength-power training produces specific strength-power adaptations (ability to perform explosive tasks), whereas aerobic training produces improvements in endurance (ability to perform sustained tasks).
- Trained muscle fibers hypertrophy, the number of mitochondria increase and the concentration of metabolic enzymes rises. Muscle capillaries proliferate, the increase being greater than that of the muscle fiber size. Consequently, diffusion distance from the oxygen source to the mitochondria is decreased and oxygen uptake improved (Starrit *et al.* 1999, Casaburi 1992).
- Body weight and fat usually decrease, whilst lean body mass increases (Casaburi 1992).
- Cardiovascular and pulmonary adaptations to endurance training optimize peripheral and central oxygen transport mechanisms (Dean 1994).
- Cardiovascular adaptations include:
  - reduction in resting and submaximal exercise heart rate;
  - increased stroke volume;
  - decreased myocardial oxygen demands;
  - increased maximal VO_2 (whole body oxygen uptake);
  - increased anaerobic threshold;
  - reduction in both systolic and diastolic blood pressure;
  - augmented blood supply to exercising muscle
  (McArdle et al 1996, Fletcher et al 1996).
- Pulmonary adaptations include:
  - increased tidal volume with reduced respiratory frequency;
  - greater oxygen extraction from the inspired air;
  - reduction in the percentage of oxygen cost attributable to breathing (McArdle et al 1996);
  - these factors may serve to reduce the sensation of exercise-induced dyspnea and increase oxygen availability for active muscle.
- Advantageous changes also occur in hormonal, hemodynamic, metabolic, antioxidant and neurological function (Powers *et al.* 1993, Fletcher *et al.* 1996).
- Exercise can also have beneficial psychological effects in terms of anxiety, depression and self-image.

Clinical relevance

- Exercise training is a key component of cardiopulmonary rehabilitation and should be of paramount importance in the physiotherapist's treatment plan. Regardless of the patient's presenting condition the fundamental principles of exercise training apply, merely administered in a manner and at a level that is appropriate for the patient's physiological reserve, condition and identified problems.
- The desired physiological adaptations are dependent upon adherence to carefully planned exercise programs. The physiotherapist must consider frequency, duration and optimal training stimulus for each patient. There is a consensus of opinion that advises training 3–5 times per week (Casaburi 1992).
- All patients should ideally have a medical assessment prior to commencing an exercise training to insure their suitability and safety.
- It is important to have a baseline patient assessment in order to monitor progress. Where possible, assessment should include an accepted exercise test, e.g. maximal/sub-maximal exercise test, walking test.
- Outcome measures are dependent upon the aims of the training program, but may include an exercise test or quality of life measure.
- Exercise training programs should be specific to the patient's requirements in terms of type of training, e.g. strength/endurance/both.
- 'Warm-up' and 'cool-down' sessions are essential to minimize the risk of cardiovascular or musculoskeletal complications.
- Where possible, the patient should be given a specific exercise prescription in terms of intensity (e.g. maximum heart rate, perceived exertion, percentage VO_{2max}, blood lactate levels), frequency and duration.
- It has been recognized that adherence to exercise programs in both healthy and symptomatic groups is often problematic. Format, supervision and location of exercise training are likely to have significant influence (Garrod 1998, CSP 1999).
- The effects of training are lost unless the exercise is continued. It is likely however that a less-intensive regime may be sufficient to maintain aerobic fitness once it has been achieved (Casaburi 1992).

Related topics

Deconditioning (p. 32); Exercise training in cardiac rehabilitation (p. 82); Exercise training in peripheral arterial obstructive disease (p. 85); Exercise training in pulmonary rehabilitation (p. 88); Mobilization (p. 113).

References and further reading

Casaburi R. (1992) Principles of exercise training. *Chest* **101**(5 Suppl): 263S–267S.
Chartered Society of Physiotherapy (1999). *Health Promotion: Physical Activity and Exercise.* Physiotherapy Effectiveness Bulletin.
Dean E. (1994) Oxygen transport: A physiologically based conceptual framework for the practice of cardiopulmonary physiotherapy. *Physiotherapy* **80**(6): 347–355.

Fletcher G.F., Balady G., Blair S.N. *et al.* (1996) Statement on exercise: Benefits and recommendations for physical activity for all Americans. *Circulation* **94**: 857–862.

Garrod R. (1998) The pros and cons of pulmonary rehabilitation at home. *Physiotherapy* **84**: 603–607.

McArdle W.D., Katch F.I. and Katch V.L. (1996) *Exercise Physiology*. 4th edition. Williams and Wilkins, Baltimore.

Powers S.K., Criswell D., Lawler J. *et al.* (1993) Rigorous exercise training increases superoxide dismutase activity in ventricular myocardium. *Am J Physiology* **256**(6pt2): H2094–2098.

Starrit E.C. (1999) Effect of short term training on mitochondrial ATP production in human skeletal muscle. *J Appl Physiol* **86**(2): 450–454.

EXERCISE TRAINING 2 – EXERCISE TRAINING IN CARDIAC REHABILITATION

Description

'The sum of the activities required to influence favourably the underlying cause of the disease, as well as the best possible physical, mental and social conditions so that they may, by their own efforts preserve or resume their proper place in society' (WHO 1993)

Key physiological principles

See also key physiological principles in Exercise Training 1.

- Lifestyle modification and risk factor avoidance contribute to both primary and secondary prevention of cardiovascular disease.
- Regular physical activity is believed to lower the risk of coronary heart disease by influencing blood pressure, lipid profile and body weight (Perk & Veress 2000).
- Total weekly exercise energy consumption of more than 2000 kcal has been suggested as a method of attenuating atherosclerosis progression (Perk & Veress 2000).
- Although exercise training has been linked to improvements in myocardial function, the increase in aerobic fitness following exercise/cardiac rehabilitation may also be attributable to improvements in the efficiency of skeletal muscle, thereby reducing myocardial work. This may be of particular importance in patients with poor left ventricular function (Humphrey & Bartels 2001).

Clinical relevance

Efficacy

- Many studies evaluating cardiac rehabilitation have included non-homogenous subjects, e.g. low-risk, middle-aged males, post-MI. Therefore any generalization of results is often difficult (Dinnes *et al.* 1999).
- A number of studies have shown that comprehensive cardiac rehabilitation improves cardiac risk factors (e.g. lipids, obesity indices, exercise capacity and adverse psychological factors), as well as significantly reducing long-term hospitalization and cardiac morbidity (Lavie & Milani 2000, Hedback *et al.* 2001).
- A systematic review indicates a reduction in cardiac mortality of up to 30%. Although exercise-based cardiac rehabilitation is effective in reducing cardiac deaths, it is not yet clear whether exercise alone or comprehensive cardiac rehabilitation is more beneficial (Jolliffe *et al.* 2001).
- Comprehensive cardiac rehabilitation is generally considered a cost-effective measure for patients with cardiac disease. However, individual program cost-

effectiveness is dependent upon factors such as location, design and patient compliance (Dinnes *et al.* 1999).

Indications for use

- Traditionally, cardiac rehabilitation has been offered to patients post-MI, angioplasty or surgical intervention. There is now increasing interest in the benefits for patients with angina or CHF and following heart transplantation (Dinnes *et al.* 1999, Humphrey & Bartels 2001).

Program design and components

- Comprehensive cardiac rehabilitation is often considered in terms of phases; in-patient recovery, out-patient rehabilitation, and long-term maintenance.
- A menu-based program is commonly offered, including exercise training, smoking cessation, dietary interventions, psychosocial support and stress management (Perk & Veress 2000).
- Although many programs are conducted in the hospital setting, some may be community or home based.

Exercise training

- Exercise training may begin in the first phase of rehabilitation, i.e. in-patient recovery. Early ambulation is advocated for patients with uncomplicated MI or cardiac surgery. The physiotherapist commonly utilizes functional activities such as walking and stair climbing. Additional intervention, e.g. management of postoperative pulmonary complications may be indicated.
- The second phase of rehabilitation commonly commences 2–6 weeks post MI, angioplasty or cardiac surgery.
- Exercise prescription must be individualized and follow the principles of intensity, frequency and duration.
- Appropriate adjustments to exercise prescription should be made for patients taking β-blockers (Eston & Connolly 1996).
- Exercise intensity may be assessed by heart rate predictive protocols, metabolic equivalents (METs) from recent stress test results, rates of perceived exertion (RPE), or resistance/speed on machinery (converted from heart rate or RPE assessment).
- Training sessions of 15–60 minutes (excluding warm-up and cool down) at 40–85% of VO_{2max}, 3–5 times weekly are commonly advocated.
- Aerobic training is often achieved with walking, cycling, stair climbing or other exercise involving large muscle mass. Upper limb exercises may also be included.
- Strength training is increasingly incorporated. It is believed to add to the effects of aerobic training by increasing muscle strength and lean body mass, and decreasing body fat (Pierson *et al.* 2001). It is believed to be safe for uncomplicated cardiac patients, even with a reduced left ventricular ejection fraction (Perk & Veress 2000). Strength training may prove to be of particular benefit to those inherently weak, e.g. CHF and heart transplant patients.
- Patient-specific physiotherapy intervention may also be appropriate, e.g. management of musculoskeletal problems, relaxation and breathing control

(c.f. ACBT, thoracic mobilization, positioning to relieve breathlessness, pain management).

Safety

- Exercise intervention has been shown to be safe with a low rate of non-fatal cardiovascular deaths (Van Camp & Peterson 1986).
- Staff must be competent in resuscitation and have appropriate equipment available, e.g. oxygen, defibrillator, GTN, etc., where it is deemed necessary.

Related topics

Deconditioning (p. 32); Exercise training 1 (p. 79); Exercise training in pulmonary rehabilitation (p. 85); Exercise training in peripheral arterial obstructive disease (p. 88); Heart failure (p. 41); Mobilization (p. 113).

References and further reading

Dinnes J., Kleijnen J., Leitner M. and Thompson D. (1999) Cardiac rehabilitation. *Quality Health Care* **8**: 65–71.

Eston R. and Connolly D. (1996) The use of ratings of perceived exertion for exercise prescription in patients receiving beta blocker therapy. *Sports Medicine* **21**: 176–190.

Hedback B., Perk J., Hornblad M. and Ohlsson U. (2001) Cardiac rehabilitation after coronary artery bypass surgery: 10-year results on morbidity, mortality and readmissions to hospital. *J Cardiovasc Risk* **8**(3): 153–158.

Humphrey R. and Bartels M.N. (2001) Exercise, cardiovascular disease and chronic heart failure. *Arch Phys Med Rehabil* **82**(Suppl 1): S76–81.

Jolliffe J.A., Rees K., Taylor R.S., Thompson D., Oldridge N. and Ebrahim N. (2001) Exercise-based rehabilitation for coronary heart disease (Cochrane Review). *Cochrane Database Syst Rev* 1: CD001800.

Lavie C.J. and Milani R.V. (2000) Benefits of cardiac rehabilitation and exercise training. *Chest* **117**(1): 5–7.

Perk J. and Veress G. (2000) Cardiac rehabilitation: applying exercise physiology in clinical practice. *Eur J Appl Physiol* **83**: 457–462.

Pierson L.M., Herbert W.G., Norton H.J., Kiebzak G.M., Griffith P., Fedor J.M., Ramp W.K. and Cook J.W. (2001) Effects of combined aerobic and resistance training versus aerobic training in cardiac rehabilitation. *J Cardiopulm Rehabil* **21**(2): 101–110.

Van Camp S.P. and Peterson R.A. (1986) Cardiovascular complications of outpatient cardiac rehabilitation programmes. *JAMA* **256**: 1160–1163.

WHO (1993) *Needs and action priorities in cardiac rehabilitation and secondary prevention in patients with coronary heart disease.* WHO Technical Report Service 831, WHO Regional Office for Europe, Geneva.

EXERCISE TRAINING 3 – EXERCISE TRAINING IN PULMONARY REHABILITATION

Description

'… a multidisciplinary program of care for patients with chronic respiratory impairment that is individually tailored and designed to optimize physical and social performance and autonomy' (American Thoracic Society 1999).

Key physiological principles

See also key physiological principles in Exercise Training 1.

- Individuals with lung disease are often extremely sedentary due to the fear of dyspnea.
- Even mild lung disease may result in muscle weakness secondary to deconditioning, hypoxia, malnutrition or sepsis (Morgan 1999). Lower limb muscles are often atrophied, and blood lactate levels elevated at very low work rates (Casaburi 1992).
- Consequently, much of the resulting disability (muscle dysfunction, cardiac impairment, skeletal disease, etc.) is attributable to the secondary effects of lung disease, rather than the disease itself (American Thoracic Society 1999).

Clinical relevance

Efficacy

- Evidence shows that a comprehensive pulmonary rehabilitation program can improve functional exercise capacity and health status, and reduce dyspnea on exertion (British Thoracic Society 2001).
- Improvements in lung function are not seen – rehabilitation appears to modify the secondary effects of the disease rather than the disease itself.
- Furthermore, incidence of reduced healthcare and pharmacological usage, and exacerbation rate have been suggested (British Thoracic Society 2001).
- Benefits of pulmonary rehabilitation have been demonstrated up to at least a year after course completion, albeit at a reduced level (Foglio *et al.* 1999). Interim 'follow-up' courses produce short-term gains, but do not appear to produce additive long-term benefits (Foglio *et al.* 2001).

Indications for use

- Patients presenting with limiting dyspnea secondary to respiratory dysfunction (approximately MRC dyspnea grade 3 – 'have to stop after 100 m', or above) (British Thoracic Society 2001).
- Pulmonary rehabilitation has traditionally been aimed at patients with CAL, however other candidates may include patients with bronchiectasis, chronic asthma, cystic fibrosis, chest wall disorders, neuromuscular disease, interstitial lung disease, or prior to lung volume reduction surgery.

- Patients must have on-going, optimal medical management, and be free from conditions that may preclude them from safe exercise, e.g. unstable angina (British Thoracic Society 2001).

Program design and components
- Pulmonary rehabilitation may be undertaken on an in- or out-patient basis. Studies show that both are equally effective, but reduced costs may indicate that out-patient rehabilitation is most efficient (British Thoracic Society 2001).
- Comprehensive pulmonary rehabilitation should incorporate exercise training, disease education, nutritional management, and cognitive behavioral intervention (Morgan 1999).
- Outcomes of rehabilitation may include measurements of exercise capacity (e.g. maximal exercise test, 6-minute walk test, shuttle walking test, ratings of perceived exertion for a given level of activity) or health status (e.g. The Chronic Respiratory Questionnaire, St. George's Respiratory Questionnaire, Breathing Problems Questionnaire) (Morgan 1999).

Exercise training and physiotherapy
- Physical training is essential in effecting the benefits associated with pulmonary rehabilitation (Morgan 1999).
- Production of the desired training effect is thought to require: course duration of 4–12 weeks, supervised 20–30 minute exercise training sessions 2–5 times per week, at a target intensity of 60–70% of VO_{2max} (British Thoracic Society 2001).
- Many patients may better tolerate interval type training alternated with rest periods. However, it is not yet clear how this may affect rehabilitation outcomes.
- Aerobic training of the lower limbs is essential, e.g. walking and/or cycling (British Thoracic Society 2001).
- Upper limb aerobic training may also be included, e.g. arm cranking to improve arm endurance.
- The addition of strength training to endurance training improves muscle bulk and power in this patient population, but has not yet been proven to further improve exercise capacity or health status (British Thoracic Society 2001).
- Conflicting evidence exists regarding ventilatory muscle training. Although inspiratory muscle training has improved the strength of inspiratory muscles in patients with CAL, it is not clear how this affects symptoms, disability or handicap (American Thoracic Society 1999). At present, ventilatory muscle training is not a common component of pulmonary rehabilitation programs (British Thoracic Society 2001, Gosselink et al. 1997).
- Exercise prescription must be regularly reviewed and progressed in terms of intensity or duration. Intensity may be set using walking speed, load or a rate of perceived exertion.
- The addition of a monitored home program to out-patient training may further improve exercise capacity (Gosselink et al. 1997).
- Patient-specific physiotherapy intervention may also be appropriate, e.g. management of musculoskeletal problems, airway clearance techniques,

relaxation and breathing control (c.f. ACBT, positioning to relieve breathlessness, pain management).

Safety

- Exercising in a 'safe' environment may also allow patients to tolerate more dyspnea than normal. This may result in a 'desensitization' effect.
- Simple first aid medication (e.g. oxygen, nebulized bronchodilators, GTN) should be available. Staff should be competent in resuscitation (British Thoracic Society 2001).
- To date, training with supplemental oxygen has not been shown to have additional effects, however it may be essential for some patients for symptomatic relief (Garrod *et al.* 2000).

Related topics

Deconditioning (p. 32); Exercise training 1 (p. 79); Exercise training in cardiac rehabilitation (p. 82); Exercise training in peripheral arterial obstructive disease (p. 88); Mobilization (p. 113).

References and further reading

American Thoracic Society (1999) Pulmonary rehabilitation. *Am J Respir Crit Care Med* **159**: 1666–1682.

British Thoracic Society Standards of Care Subcommittee on Pulmonary Rehabilitation (2001) Pulmonary rehabilitation. *Thorax* **56**: 827–834.

Casaburi R. (1992) Principles of exercise training. *Chest* **101**(5 Suppl): 263S–267S.

Foglio K., Bianchi L., Bruletti G., Battista L., Pagani M. and Ambrosino N. (1999) Long term effectiveness of pulmonary rehabilitation in patients with chronic airway obstruction. *Eur Respir J* **13**(1): 125–132.

Foglio K., Bianchi L. and Ambrosino N. (2001) Is it really useful to repeat out-patient pulmonary rehabilitation programs in patients with chronic airway obstruction? A 2-year controlled study. *Chest* **119**(6): 1696–1704.

Garrod R., Paul E.A. and Wedzicha J.A. (2000) Supplemental oxygen during pulmonary rehabilitation in patients with COAD with exercise hypoxaemia. *Thorax* **55**(7): 539–543.

Gosselink R., Troosters T. and Decramer M. (1997) Exercise training in COPD patients: the basic questions. *Eur Respir J* **10**(12): 2884–2891.

Morgan M.D.L. (1999) The prediction of benefit from pulmonary rehabilitation: setting, training intensity and the effect of selection by disability. *Thorax* **54**(Suppl 2): S3–7.

EXERCISE TRAINING 4 – EXERCISE TRAINING IN PERIPHERAL ARTERIAL OBSTRUCTIVE DISEASE (PAOD)

Description

The use of specifically designed exercise training regimes for patients with intermittent claudication.

Key physiological principles

See also key physiological principles in Exercise Training 1.

- Reduced exercise capacity in patients with PAOD is not solely due to reduced lower limb blood flow.
- Contributing factors include:
  – metabolic inefficiency;
  – diminished cardio-respiratory reserve;
  – exercise induced inflammation
  (Tan *et al.* 2000).
- Although exercise training has not consistently been shown to increase blood flow to the lower extremity, other possible mechanisms for improvement include redistribution of blood flow and improved oxidative capacity of the muscles (Tan *et al.* 2000).
- Improvements may also be seen in blood rheology and cardiopulmonary function (Tan *et al.* 2000).

Clinical relevance

Efficacy

- Exercise training was first shown to be an effective method of improving symptoms of claudication in a randomized controlled trial in 1966 (cited by Hunt *et al.* 1999).
- A systematic review of 10 well-executed trials concluded that exercise is of significant benefit to patients with leg pain on walking (Leng *et al.* 2000).
- Exercise therapy was associated with improvements in maximal walking time and walking ability. Furthermore, exercise produced significant improvements in walking time compared with both angioplasty at 6 months and anti-platelet therapy, and did not differ significantly from surgical treatment (Leng *et al.* 2000).
- The development/validation of a disease-specific instrument for the assessment of symptomatic outcome for patients with intermittent claudication is required.

Indications for use

- To date, studies have not identified predictive factors for the outcomes of exercise therapy in intermittent claudication. Consequently, selection of patients who are most likely to benefit is arbitrary (Robeer *et al.* 1998).

Exercise training

- Exercise therapy should be conducted at least three times per week at near maximal claudication pain (Leng 1999).
- The program targets those muscles which become ischemic during exercise, thus allowing adaptations to occur (Gardner & Poehlman 1995).
- Exercise-induced gain is lost when training is discontinued, therefore, methods of long-term support should be investigated (Hunt *et al.* 1999).
- Long-term benefits of exercise in this group of patients also require clarification (CSP 1999).

Safety

- Staff must be competent in resuscitation and have appropriate equipment available (e.g. oxygen, defibrillator, GTN, etc.) where it is deemed necessary.

Related topics

Deconditioning (p. 32); Exercise training 1 (p. 79); Exercise training in cardiac rehabilitation (p. 82); Exercise training in pulmonary rehabilitation (p. 85); Mobilization (p. 113).

References and further reading

Chartered Society of Physiotherapy (1999) *Health Promotion: Physical Activity and Exercise.* Physiotherapy Effectiveness Bulletin.

Gardner A. and Poehlman E. (1995) Exercise rehabilitation programs for the treatment of claudication pain. *JAMA* 27: 975–980.

Hunt D., Leighton M. and Reed G. (1999) Intermittent claudication: implementation of an exercise programme. *Physiotherapy* 85: 149–153.

Leng G.C., Fowler B. and Ernst E. (2000) Exercise for intermittent claudication. *Cochrane Database Syst Rev* (2): CD000990.

Robeer G.G., Brandsma J.W., van den Heuvel S.P., Smit B., Oostendorp R.A. and Wittens C.H. (1998) Exercise therapy for intermittent claudication: A review of the quality of randomised controlled trials and evaluation of predictive factors. *Eur J Vasc Endovasc Surg* 15(1): 36–43.

Tan K.H., De Cossart L. and Edwards P.R. (2000) Exercise training and peripheral vascular disease. *Br J Surg* 87(5): 553–562.

FLUTTER

Description

A small mechanical device that incorporates a high-density ball bearing. Expiratory airflow moves the ball bearing producing both positive expiratory pressure (PEP) and high frequency oscillations of air within the airways.

Key physiological principles

- The production of PEP increases end-expiratory lung volume thereby reducing airway resistance and small airway closure (West 1995).
- Channels of collateral ventilation are recruited allowing air to flow behind sputum plugs, facilitating secretion movement.
- It is claimed that the Flutter device generates sufficient PEP to produce these effects, and in addition, the high-frequency oscillations generated by the flutter create airway vibrations that mobilize excess secretions.

Clinical relevance

Efficacy

- It is claimed that Flutter can generate PEP of 10–20 cmH_2O in the airways. However, there have been no trials to support this.
- It has been proposed that the high-frequency oscillations aid secretion clearance. Freitag *et al.* (1989) suggested that such oscillations might not mobilize secretions in the right direction. However, others suggest that the oscillatory effect may be responsible for reducing sputum viscoelasticity (App *et al.* 1998).
- Flutter combined with spontaneous coughing has been shown to be less effective than ACBT (Pryor *et al.* 1994). However, Flutter combined with FET should improve effectiveness (Pryor 1999) (c.f. ACBT).
- The use of Flutter in patients with CF has been reported to increase sputum yield compared to two other regimes (GAP and spontaneous coughing). However, it should be noted that clinically these two regimes would not be used in isolation (c.f. GAP).
- For effective use the Flutter should ideally be kept in a position perpendicular to the mouth. This may make its use less effective in some GAP.

Indications for use

- The use of Flutter may improve adherence with self-management regimes.
- The Flutter can be useful in the treatment of children.

Related topics

Altered respiratory compliance (p. 23); Impaired tracheobronchial clearance (p. 48); Reduced lung volume (p. 61).

References and further reading

App E.M., Kieselmann R., Reinhardt D., Lindemann H., Dasgupta B., King M. and Brand P. (1998) Sputum rheology changes in CF lung disease following 2 different types of physiotherapy: Flutter vs autogenic drainage. *Chest* **114**(1): 171–177.

Freitag L., Bremme J. and Schroer M. (1989) High frequency oscillation for respiratory physiotherapy. *Br J Anaes* **63**: 44s–46s.

Pryor J.A. (1999) Physiotherapy for airway clearance in adults. *Eur Respir J* **14**: 1418–1424.

Pryor J., Webber B., Hodson M. and Warner J. (1994) The Flutter VRP1 as an adjunct to chest physiotherapy in CF. *Respir Med* **88**: 677–681.

West J. (1995) *Respiratory Physiology*, 5th edition. Williams & Wilkins, Baltimore.

GLOSSOPHARYNGEAL BREATHING

Description

Glossopharyngeal breathing (GPB) is a voluntary technique whereby the patient 'gulps' boluses of air into the lungs.

Key physiological principles

- GPB constitutes a form of positive pressure ventilation, augmenting vital capacity.
- It may assist ventilation and effective coughing or speech (Dail & Affeldt 1955).

Clinical relevance

Efficacy

- It has been found that patients with poliomyelitis were able to use GPB at a rate of 60 to 200 times per minute.
- 700–1000 ml of air could be added to the patient's vital capacity following 10–20 gulps of air (c.f. reduced lung volumes).
- Metcalfe (1966) found that vital capacity could be increased from 60% to 81% of its predicted value when using GPB.
- The use of GPB has been shown to be sufficient to maintain arterial blood gases within normal range (Affeldt *et al.* 1955) (c.f. acid–base disturbances).
- Affeldt *et al.* (1955) discovered that a patient's proficiency at GPB was independent of the extent of muscle paralysis (c.f. respiratory muscle dysfunction).
- The ability to perform GPB is dependent upon effective activity of the lips, mouth, tongue, soft palate, pharynx and larynx (Pryor & Webber 1998).
- Ardran *et al.* (1959) discovered that patients with palatal and laryngeal weakness, could sometimes be taught GPB if a nose clip was used.
- A successful outcome is dependent upon a good technique. GPB is often both difficult to master and time consuming to teach.

Indications for use

- GPB was first described as a trick movement seen in patients with poliomyelitis (Dail 1951).
- GPB is an effective maneuver to augment tidal volume in any patient who is unable to voluntarily alter tidal breathing.
- Dail & Affeldt (1955) taught GPB to 100 patients with poliomyelitis. They found that 69 patients used this technique to assist normal breathing and 31 to assist speech and coughing. 42 patients found that GPB allowed them to discontinue respiratory support (c.f. mechanical ventilation, NIPPV).
- GPB may prove useful in improving cough effectiveness in patients with tetraplegia or neuromuscular disorders (Pryor 1999) (c.f. impaired tracheobronchial clearance).

Contraindications

- GPB is contraindicated in patients with a tracheostomy when the cuff is inflated.
- GPB must be avoided in patients with airflow obstruction or pulmonary disease, due to the risk of air trapping.

Related topics

Impaired gaseous exchange (p. 44); Impaired tracheobronchial clearance (p. 48); Reduced lung volume (p. 61).

References and further reading

Affeldt J.E., Dail C.W., Collier C.R. and Farr A.F. (1955) Glossopharyngeal breathing: ventilation studies. *J Appl Physiol* **8**: 11–13.

Ardran G.M., Kelleher W.H. and Kemp F.H. (1959) Cineradiographic studies of glossopharyngeal breathing. *Br J Radiog* **32**: 322–328.

Dail C.W. (1951) Glossopharyngeal breathing by paralysed patients. *California Med* **75**: 217–218.

Dail C.W. and Affeldt J.E. (1955) Clinical aspects of glossopharyngeal breathing. *JAMA* **158**: 445–449.

Metcalfe V.A. (1966) Vital capacity and glossopharyngeal breathing in traumatic quadriplegia. *Phys Ther* **46**: 835–838.

Pryor J.A. (1999) Physiotherapy for airway clearance in adults. *Euro Respir J* **14**(6): 1418–1424.

Pryor J.A. and Webber B.A. (1998) *Physiotherapy for Respiratory and Cardiac Problems*, 2nd edition. Churchill Livingstone, Edinburgh.

HUMIDIFICATION

Description

Humidification of dry gas may be achieved by inhalation of a vapor, inhalation of an aerosol or by heat and moisture exchange.

Key physiological principles

Inspired gas is normally heated and humidified via the nose and upper airways, the nasal septum and turbinates that increase the mucosal surface area available for evaporation. Consequences of inadequate heating/humidification include:

- dehydration/damage of the cilia;
- facilitation of bacterial colonization;
- alteration of the periciliary fluid;
- defective mucus rheology;
- impaired mucociliary clearance
  (Fowler 2000, Hedley & Allt-Graham 1994).

Clinical relevance

Efficacy

- The 'beneficial' effect of humidification, i.e. improved mucociliary clearance, is often attributed to repletion of the periciliary fluid and reduction in mucus viscosity by absorption of the solution into the gel layer (c.f. impaired tracheobronchial clearance).
- Cough efficiency is thought to improve as mucus viscosity decreases and periciliary fluid increases (to an optimal level). Tracheobronchial clearance is accelerated when humidification is used as an adjunct to physiotherapy in bronchiectatic subjects (Conway 1992).
- To date, the benefits of water or isotonic saline solution humidification for self-ventilating patients with an intact upper respiratory tract remain unproven.
- Nebulized *hypertonic* saline solutions have been shown to accelerate mucociliary clearance (Wark & McDonald 2000). This effect is usually attributed to a rheological alteration in the sputum allowing improved transportation by the cilia. This effect is exploited during sputum induction, but any other therapeutic significance is unproven.
- Heat and moisture exchangers (HME) incorporating filter systems can provide physiological levels of humidity and reduce the risk of cross infection, in the patient whose upper airway has been bypassed. This method of humidification may therefore be extremely cost-effective in terms of decreased patient morbidity, equipment and labor intensity.
- The moisture output of HME declines with increasing tidal and minute volumes, and consequently may be implicated in development of tenacious

secretions or tracheal tube occlusion (Hedley & Allt-Graham 1994) (c.f. tracheostomy management).

Indications for use

- Humidification is not a replacement for adequate systemic hydration.
- If the normal humidification system is bypassed with a tracheostomy or endotracheal tube supplemental humidification is required.
- A humidification system is also indicated when using mechanical aids with high-flow delivery of dry gas, e.g. CPAP or MV.
- Humidification may be considered when oxygen flow rate is >4 l/min (Bateman & Leach 1998).
- Anecdotal reports support the use of humidification for patients with tenacious secretions (especially with co-existing infection) to facilitate mucociliary clearance (c.f. impaired tracheobronchial clearance).
- Humidification is not usually necessary for patients with long-term, permanent tracheostomies as the airway epithelium adapts accordingly.

Administration

- Heated water bath systems deliver humidity as a vapor. The efficiency of vapor production is improved by increasing the temperature of the solution to approximately 36–38°C. These systems are most commonly used in the intubated patient or those receiving high-flow, dry gas.
- Jet nebulizers or ultrasonic nebulizers deliver humidity as an aerosol. Many types of large volume jet nebulization systems are available for single patient use, some incorporating heating devices. Ultrasonic nebulizers have significantly higher rates of solution production.
- HME are disposable devices that conserve both heat and moisture from exhaled breath, allowing heating and humidification of the inhaled breath. The principles of heat and moisture exchange are exploited in a variety of devices designed for use in ventilator circuits or with tracheostomies.
- Developments of the HME system have been described which add external heat and water at the patient side of the HME (Larsson *et al.* 2000).
- Particle size should be considered when selecting humidification devices. A therapeutic range should be sought with a lower range of 2 μm.
- Humidification devices designed to be used in conjunction with narrow bore tubing are less clinically effective and therefore not recommended.
- Humidification should not be used in conjunction with venturi valve systems, as moisture within the valve will affect the FiO_2.
- Humidification is not necessary with nasal cannulae as the oxygen flow rate should always be 4 l/min or less.
- Sterile water is the most commonly used humidification solution, with selective use of isotonic or hypertonic saline.

Cautions and complications

- In patients with hyper-reactive airways, bronchospasm may be associated with unheated humidification, ultrasonic nebulization or use of an agent other than isotonic saline.

- Hypertonic saline should be used in a supervised area where appropriate resuscitation may be performed if required.
- Devices containing a water reservoir may be rapidly colonized, particularly with Gram-negative bacteria such as *Pseudomonas* (Hedley & Allt-Graham 1994). Where possible, the system should be sterile.
- Burns have been reported with faulty heated systems. A cut-out device should always be used and the equipment appropriately maintained.
- Although slight, the risk of over humidification should be considered, e.g. in patients with marked pulmonary edema. The effects of over humidification include increased secretions, atelectasis and subsequent hypoxemia.
- Under humidification may result in obstructed or occluded tracheostomy or endotracheal tubes. Consequently, the adequacy of the selected humidification system must be regularly assessed.

Related topics

Effects of general anesthesia (p. 39); Impaired tracheobronchial clearance (p. 48); Tracheostomy management (p. 148); Oxygen therapy (p. 118).

References and further reading

Bateman N.T. and Leach R.M. (1998) ABC of oxygen: Acute oxygen therapy. *BMJ* 317 (7161): 798–801.

Conway J.H. (1992) The effects of humidification for patients with chronic airways disease. *Physiotherapy* 78(2): 97–101.

Fowler S. (2000) A guide to humidification. *Nursing Times*, May 18.

Hedley R.M. and Allt-Graham J. (1994) Heat and moisture exchangers and breathing filters. *Br J Anaes* 73: 227–236.

Larsson A., Gustafsson A. and Svanborg L. (2000) A new device for the 100 per cent humidification of inspired air. *Crit Care* 4(1): 54–60.

Peterson B.D. (1968) Heated humidifiers: structure and function. *Respir Care Clin North Am* 4(2): 243–259.

Wark P.A. and McDonald V. (2000) Nebulised hypertonic saline for CF. *Cochrane Database Syst Rev* (2): CD001506.

Williams R., Rankin N., Smith T., Galler D. and Seakins P. (1996) Relationship between the humidity and temperature of inspired gas and the function of the airway mucosa. *Crit Care Med* 24(11): 1920–1929.

INCENTIVE SPIROMETRY (IS)

Description

Mechanical devices (flow or volume sensitive) intended to emphasize an inspiratory maneuver by providing visual feedback.

Key physiological principles

- IS is designed to provide the patient with visual motivation to optomize tidal volume or inspiratory flow rate.
- The physiological benefits are those associated with an augmented tidal volume or slow, sustained inspiratory flow, e.g. enhancing interdependence, reducing resistance to flow and recruiting collateral ventilation.

Clinical relevance

Efficacy

- IS has been extensively studied; compared with IPPB, CPAP, 'chest physiotherapy', early mobilization, deep breathing, PEP, and various combinations of the above. Many studies have failed to show any conclusive benefit of IS over other techniques.
- Current evidence does not support the use of incentive spirometry in the prevention of postoperative pulmonary complications following cardiac or upper abdominal surgery (Overend *et al.* 2001). However, incentive spirometry and deep breathing exercises are more effective than no physiotherapy intervention in the prevention of pulmonary complications following upper abdominal surgery (Thomas and McIntosh 1994).
- Lederer *et al.* (1980) discovered that despite IS education and availability at the bedside, a substantial number of patients did not independently use the device in the postoperative period.
- Furthermore, Van de Water (1980) revealed that encouragement to deep breathe by hospital personnel was superior to IS in restoring pulmonary function.

Indications for use

- Proponents of IS maintain that it functions as an 'aide memoir' to treatment.
- In the management of a pediatric patient the use of IS may be introduced as a game. This may improve compliance with treatment.

Related topics

Effects of general anesthesia (p. 39); Impaired gaseous exchange (p. 44); Impaired tracheobronchial clearance (p. 48); Reduced lung volume (p. 61).

References and further reading

Lederer D.H., Van de Water J.M. and Indech R.B. (1980) Which deep breathing device should the post-operative patient use? *Chest* 77: 610–613.

Overend T.J., Anderson C.M., Lucy S.D., Bhatia C., Jonsson B.I. and Timmermans C. (2001) The effect of incentive spirometry on postoperative complications: a systematic review. *Chest* **120**(3): 971–978.

Thomas J.A. and McIntosh J.M. (1994) Are incentive spirometry, IPPB and deep breathing exercises effective in the prevention of post-operative pulmonary complications after upper abdominal surgery? A systematic overview and meta-analysis. *Physical Therapy* 74(1): 3–10.

Van de Water J.M. (1980) Pre-operative and post-operative techniques in the prevention of pulmonary complications. *Surg Clin North Am* **60**: 1339–1348.

INTERMITTENT POSITIVE PRESSURE BREATHING (IPPB)

Description

Use of a pressure limited respirator to apply positive inspiratory pressure (with aerosol). Gas flow is triggered by the spontaneous effort of the patient. Flow continues until a pre-set pressure has been attained, and then expiration is passive.

Key physiological principles

- When IPPB is applied to a relaxed and appropriately positioned patient, tidal volume and minute volume are augmented, increasing the rate of alveolar ventilation. This produces an increase in P_aO_2, and a decrease in P_aCO_2.
- By applying positive pressure to the airway in this manner, IPPB aims to reduce the 'demand' side of the work of breathing equation. (Bott *et al.* 1992).

Clinical relevance

Efficacy

- Despite the widespread use of IPPB, controversy has arisen because of a number of conflicting and questionable trials (Bott *et al.* 1992). However, clinically the use of IPPB has proved to be a valuable adjunct to physiotherapy treatment.
- IPPB has been shown to increase ventilation, improve arterial blood gases and reduce work of breathing when the patient is relaxed and positioned appropriately (Denehy & Berney 2001).
- IPPB passively augments tidal volume, and therefore may reduce resistance to airflow, enhance interdependence and thus aid in re-expansion of alveoli with sputum-related collapse. However, used in isolation, it will have no effect on FRC (c.f. reduced lung volumes).
- The effects of IPPB are relatively short-lived lasting less than 1 hour after treatment (AARC 1993).
- Spontaneous deep breaths and IPPB are equally effective at increasing the transpulmonary pressure gradient. Therefore, IPPB should only be applied where clinically indicated.
- By increasing tidal volume, cough effectiveness may be improved and airway clearance enhanced. It has also been postulated that use of a slow inspiratory flow rate may enhance 2-phase flow (c.f. impaired tracheobronchial clearance).
- Clinically, it is more likely that a combination of techniques, e.g. IPPB with GAP, ACBT and/or manual techniques applied to the chest wall, will be most effective in promoting secretion clearance (Denehy & Berney 2001) (c.f. ACBT, GAP, manual techniques).
- Studies examining the role of IPPB during an acute exacerbation of CAL have provided conflicting results. A study of subjects with a high ventilatory demand showed that IPPB increased inspiratory muscle work and discomfort (Mancebo *et al.* 1995). However, this can be minimized by careful adjustment of the respirator settings.

- IPPB has not been demonstrated to be of use in stable CAL patients (IPPB trial group 1983).
- Studies to date have failed to show any added benefit of IPPB over 'conventional physiotherapy' in the management of *routine* postoperative patients, who can spontaneously deep breathe and have an effective cough.
- IPPB as a drug delivery device, has been shown to be as effective as a nebulizer (AARC 1993).

Indications for use

- IPPB may be of benefit to patients who hypoventilate (and/or retain bronchial secretions) secondary to fatigue, weakness or diminished consciousness.
- IPPB has been advocated for patients with altered respiratory compliance, e.g. secondary to kyphoscoliosis, neuromuscular disease and atelectasis.
- Further investigation regarding the use of IPPB to increase respiratory compliance in specific patient groups is warranted.

Patient positioning and use

- IPPB can be delivered via a mouthpiece, flange, nasal or full facemask. A full facemask may be essential in patients with diminished level of consciousness.
- Accurate positioning is essential for the effective use of IPPB. The absence of normal diaphragmatic activity results in a greater distribution of the inspired gas to nondependent regions (Chevrolet *et al.* 1978).
- As IPPB respirators are pressure cycled, less inspired gas will be distributed to areas of low compliance. Consequently, greater pressures are required to achieve a given tidal volume when lung compliance is low (Oikkonen *et al.* 1991).
- To obtain optimal distribution of inspired gas, the flow rate should ideally be slow, however, the patient may require a higher flow rate particularly if dyspneic or after expectorating.
- Peak inspiratory pressure and trigger sensitivity should be selected and carefully adjusted according to the judgment of the therapist following a thorough assessment.
- IPPB respirators used with gas flow provided from a central 'wall-mounted' source will deliver 30–40% oxygen, depending on the flow rate selected (c.f. oxygen therapy & humidification).
- IPPB respirators can be connected to an air cylinder for the treatment of patients with a 'hypoxic drive'. In this case low-flow oxygen via nasal specs or facemask should be kept at hand to provide oxygenation in between breathing cycles.

Contraindications

- The only absolute contraindication for IPPB use is an undrained pneumothorax. Otherwise the physiotherapist must assess the patient, and proceed cautiously with those who are likely to have reduced tolerance of positive pressure breathing (AARC 1993).

Related topics

Altered respiratory compliance (p. 23); Derangements in acid–base balance (p. 17); Impaired gaseous exchange (p. 44); Impaired tracheobronchial clearance (p. 48); Reduced lung volume (p. 61); Respiratory failure (p. 63); Ventilation/perfusion mismatch (p. 136).

References and further reading

AARC Clinical Practice Guideline IPPB (1993) *Respir Care* **38**(11): 1189–1195.

Bott J., Keilty S. and Noone L. (1992) IPPB – a dying art? *Physiotherapy* **78**(9): 656–660.

Chevrolet J., Martin J., Flood R., Martin R. and Engel L. (1978) Topographical ventilation and perfusion distribution during IPPB in the lateral posture. *Am Rev Respir Dis* **118**: 847–853.

Denehy L. and Berney S. (2001) The use of positive pressure devices by physiotherapists. *Eur Respir J* **17**: 821–829.

IPPB Trial Group (1983) IPPB therapy of chronic pulmonary disease – a clinical trial. *Ann Intern Med* **99**: 612–620.

Mancebo J., Isabey D., Lorino H., Lofaso F., Lemaire F. and Brochard L. (1995) Comparative effects of pressure support ventilation and IPPB in non-intubated healthy subjects. *Euro Respir J* **8**: 1901–1909.

Oikkonen M., Karjalainen K., Kahara V., Kuosa R. and Schavikin L. (1991) Comparison of incentive spirometry and IPPB after coronary artery bypass graft. *Chest* **99**: 60–65.

MANUAL HYPERINFLATION (MHI)

Description

MHI is the manual inflation of the lungs of intubated or tracheotomized patients. A volume approximately 50% greater than the baseline tidal volume is given, usually with an augmented FiO_2. The technique is administered using a re-breathing or self-inflating circuit.

Key physiological principles

In the presence of disease and/or intubation, flow-related atelectasis (e.g. sputum retention) and/or volume-related atelectasis (e.g. hypoventilation) may occur, reducing lung compliance and adversely affecting ventilation–perfusion relationships (Nunn 1993). The reported beneficial effects of MHI have been attributed to:

- Increasing expiratory airflow velocity favors 2-phase flow (c.f. impaired tracheobronchial clearance), thereby aiding airway clearance. This may be further enhanced by the application of additional techniques, e.g. GAP and chest wall vibrations.
- Delivery of an augmented tidal volume reduces the resistance to airflow and enhances interdependence, and therefore it has been postulated that MHI may recruit atelactatic lung (Denehy 1999) (c.f. reduced lung volumes, altered respiratory compliance).

Clinical relevance

Efficacy

- Many studies have produced conflicting results regarding the clinical effects of MHI, e.g. changes in lung compliance, gas exchange, atelectasis and hemo-dynamic status. Continuing research to elucidate reliability, safety and efficacy of the technique is recommended (Denehy 1999).
- The addition of MHI (peak airway pressure of 40 cmH_2O, sustained for not less than 2 seconds) to physiotherapy treatment of positioning and suctioning in mechanically ventilated patients produced improvements in respiratory compliance and sputum clearance in a small, multicenter randomized controlled trial (c.f. impaired tracheobronchial clearance). These effects were achieved without compromise of gas exchange or hemodynamics (Hodgson *et al.* 2000).
- Periodic inflations to pressures of 30–40 cmH_2O have been shown to effect alveolar recruitment, reversing induced atelectasis in normal subjects (Rothen *et al.* 1993). However, clinicians may limit peak airway pressures in order to minimize the risk of lung injury, and therefore fail to attain 'therapeutic' levels.
- Some studies have explored the effects of 'recruitment maneuvers', predominantly in animal models of acute lung injury. These sustained inflations (transpulmonary pressure of 30 cmH_2O, PEEP > closing pressure, application

of 20–40 seconds) are postulated to improve lung compliance and reduce the level of PEEP necessary to sustain open lung (Rimensberger *et al.* 1999) (c.f. altered respiratory compliance). Recruitment maneuvers in humans must be convincingly demonstrated before such practice is adopted.

- Administration of 100% oxygen, delivered at a volume 1.5 times greater than the baseline via MHI is known to be effective in preventing adverse responses to suction (Goodnough 1985) (c.f. suction).

Application of MHI

- The number of 'hyperinflation' breaths administered during treatment is highly variable, depending on patient response.
- A slow sustained inspiration during MHI minimizes peak inspiratory pressure and is associated with a more homogenous distribution of gas.
- A quick release expiratory phase enhances expiratory flow rate and therefore secretion removal (McCarren & Chow 1996).

Precautions

- Hemodynamic variables should be continually and vigilantly monitored during MHI, as significant and sustained falls in cardiac output may occur.
- The hemodynamic response to MHI will be influenced by many factors including hypovolemia, sepsis, certain pharmacological agents, cardiac dysfunction and spinal injury.
- Techniques that increase intrathoracic pressure or deliver a large tidal volume, have been implicated in lung injury (c.f. mechanical ventilation). However, there is currently no documented evidence reporting lung injury secondary to MHI in the clinical setting (McCarren & Chow 1996).
- It is advised that in order to perform safe and effective MHI, delivered pressures and/or volumes should be monitored (Robson 1998).
- Quick, sharp inflations intended to stimulate a cough are associated with high-airway pressures, and may be detrimental (c.f. impaired tracheobronchial clearance).
- In 1991 a questionnaire revealed that only 6% of physiotherapists used a PEEP valve in the MHI circuit when patients were ventilated with PEEP (King & Morrell 1991). Repeated loss of PEEP results in 'de-recruitment' (collapse) in unstable alveoli. Damaging shear forces are associated with continued alveolar reopening following collapse. It is recommended that a PEEP valve is incorporated into the circuit when indicated (Robson 1998).

Contraindications

- Where possible, alternatives to MHI (and therefore ventilator disconnection) should be sought for patients who are extremely PEEP dependent and/or requiring maximal ventilatory support.
- The use of MHI is contraindicated in the presence of unexplained hemoptysis, severe bronchospasm or an undrained pneumothorax. In situations where a pneumothorax has been treated with an effective chest drain, MHI is permitted but may be less effective.

- MHI is generally contraindicated in patients with raised intracranial pressure (ICP) (Gerard & Bullock 1986). However, in the presence of significant lung collapse or retained secretions, physiotherapy treatment including MHI, may be indicated. When using MHI in these patients, small fast breaths should be interspersed between hyperinflations to prevent a rise in P_aCO_2.

Related topics

Altered respiratory compliance (p. 23); Impaired gaseous exchange (p. 44); Impaired tracheobronchial clearance (p. 48); Reduced lung volume (p. 61).

References and further reading

Denehy L. (1999) The use of manual hyperinflation in airway clearance. *Eur Respir J* 14: 958–965.

Gerard J. and Bullock M. (1986) The effect of respiratory therapy on intracranial pressure in ventilated neurosurgical patients. *Aust J Physiother* 32: 107–111.

Goodnough S.K.C. (1985) The effects of oxygen and hyperinflation on arterial oxygen tension after endotracheal suctioning. *Heart Lung* 14: 11–17.

Hodgson C., Denehy L., Ntoumenopoulos G., Santamaria J. and Carroll S. (2000) An investigation of the early effects of manual lung hyperinflation in critically ill patients. *Anaesth Intensive Care* 28(3): 255–261.

King D. and Morrell A. (1991) A survey on manual hyperinflation as a physiotherapy technique in intensive care units. *Physiotherapy* 78: 747–750.

McCarren B. and Chow C. (1996) Manual hyperinflation: a description of the technique. *Aust J Physiotherapy* 42: 203–208.

Nunn J.F. (1993) *Nunn's Applied Respiratory Physiology*, 4th edition. Butterworth Heinemann, Oxford.

Rimensberger P.C., Pristine G., Mullen B.M., Cox P.N. and Slutsky A.S. (1999) Lung recruitment during small tidal volume ventilation allows minimal PEEP without augmenting lung injury. *Crit Care Med* 27(9): 1940–1952.

Robson W.P. (1998) To bag or not to bag? Manual hyperinflation in intensive care. *Intensive Crit Care Nurs* 14(5): 239–243.

Rothen H., Sporre B., Engberg G., Wegenius G. and Hedstierna G. (1993) Re-expansion of atelectasis during general anaesthesia: a computed tomography study. *Br J Anaesthesia* 71: 788–795.

MANUAL TECHNIQUES 1 – CHEST CLAPPING/PERCUSSION

Description

Rhythmical flexion/extension from the shoulders and elbow with a relaxed wrist and a cupped hand, applied over a patient's thorax. Can be performed single or double handed for use in adults. In pediatrics, clapping can be applied with two or three fingertips for the same effect.

Key physiological principles

- It was originally thought that chest clapping would produce a mechanical oscillation transmitted through the chest wall, to assist the mobilization of secretions. However, there is no evidence to support this statement.
- Mechanical percussion has been shown to increase intrathoracic pressure (Flower *et al.* 1979) and a similar effect may occur during chest clapping. However, the relationship between this pressure increase and airway clearance is yet to be established (Pryor 1999).

Clinical relevance

Efficacy

- Chest clapping is effective in stimulating a cough in children, young infants and babies who are unable to participate in active breathing techniques (Pryor & Webber 1998). This is due to increased chest wall compliance.
- A higher rate of chest clapping is more effective in terms of sputum clearance than a slower rate (Gallon 1991).
- Evidence shows that chest clapping added additional benefit to lower thoracic expansion exercises (c.f. ACBT) in a group of stable patients with cystic fibrosis (Webber *et al.* 1985).
- Slow one-handed chest clapping has been shown to reduce intracranial pressure in ventilated, neurosurgical patients (Parataz & Burns 1993).

Indications for use

- Patients have reported that chest clapping is a useful adjunct to treatment both when clinically stable and during acute exacerbations (Carr *et al.* 1995).

Precautions

- When used in isolation, chest clapping has been shown to cause increased airway obstruction (Wollmer *et al.* 1985). However, when used in conjunction with the ACBT no additional airflow obstruction has been found (Pryor & Webber 1979).
- Vigourous chest clapping may induce bronchospasm in patients with hyper-responsive airways (Pryor & Webber 1998) (c.f. airflow limitation).

- Prolonged chest clapping may produce hypoxemia (McDonnell *et al.* 1986). However, when used in short duration, less than 30 seconds, together with thoracic expansion exercises, no fall in oxygenation is seen (Pryor *et al.* 1990).

Contraindications
- Manual techniques should not be considered in the presence of frank hemoptysis, over unstable fractures or severe osteoporosis.

Related topics

Impaired gaseous exchange (p. 44); Impaired tracheobronchial clearance (p. 48).

References and further reading

Carr L., Pryor J.A. and Hodson M.E. (1995) Self-chest clapping: patients' views and the effects on oxygen saturation. *Physiotherapy* **81**: 753–757.

Flower K.A., Eden R.I., Lomax L., Mann N.M. and Burgess J. (1979) New mechanical aid to physiotherapy in cystic fibrosis. *BMJ* **2**: 630–631.

Gallon A. (1991) Evaluation of chest percussion in the treatment of patients with copious sputum production. *Respir Med* **85**(1): 45–51.

McDonnell T., McNicholas W.T. and Fitzgerald M.X. (1986) Hypoxaemia in chest physiotherapy in patients with cystic fibrosis. *Irish J Med Sci* **155**: 345–348.

Parataz J. and Burns Y. (1993) The effect of respiratory physiotherapy on intracranial pressure, mean arterial pressure, cerebral perfusion pressure and end-tidal carbon dioxide in ventilated neurosurgical patients. *Physio Theory Practice* **9**: 3–11.

Pryor J.A. (1999) Physiotherapy for airway clearance in adults. *Eur Respir J* **14**: 1418–1424.

Pryor J.A. and Webber B.A. (1979) An evaluation of the forced expiration technique as an adjunct to postural drainage. *Physiotherapy* **65**: 304–307.

Pryor J.A. and Webber B.A. (1998) *Physiotherapy for Respiratory and Cardiac Problems*, 2nd edition. Churchill Livingstone, Edinburgh.

Pryor J.A., Webber B.A. and Hodson M.E. (1990) Effect of chest physiotherapy on oxygen saturation in patients with cystic fibrosis. *Thorax* **45**: 77.

Webber B.A., Parker R., Hofmeyr J. and Modson M.E. (1985) Evaluation of self-percussion during postural drainage using the forced expiration technique. *Physiotherapy Practice* **1**: 42–45.

Wollmer P., Ursing K., Midgren B. and Eriksson L. (1985) Inefficiency of chest percussion in the physical therapy of chronic bronchitis. *Euro J Respir Dis* **66**: 233–239.

MANUAL TECHNIQUES 2 – CHEST SHAKING, VIBRATIONS AND COMPRESSION

Description

Chest shaking is the manual application of a vibratory force through the chest wall during the expiratory phase of the respiratory cycle. When it is performed with a coarse motion it is called chest shaking (approximately 2 Hz), and a fine motion is called vibration (approximately 12–20 Hz). Compression is the manual application of a sustained pressure to the thorax during huffing or coughing.

Key physiological principles

- Chest shaking and vibrations are based on the principle of increased expiratory airflow secondary to transmitted oscillations through the chest wall.
- It is postulated that this increase in expiratory airflow velocity may aid airway clearance by favoring 2-phase flow (c.f. impaired tracheobronchial clearance) and stimulating a cough. However, there is little scientific evidence to support this claim.

Clinical relevance

- Anecdotally, chest shaking, vibrations and compression appear to assist in the removal of excess bronchial secretions.
- Clinically, it is often a useful adjunct to stimulate a cough reflex.
- There is no standardization in the application of these techniques, making evaluation of clinical relevance difficult.

Efficacy

- In the treatment of the paralysed patient, Braun *et al.* (1984) recorded a 15% increase in peak expiratory flow, during the application of chest compression to the lower thorax.
- Chest shaking and vibrations are often used clinically during the expiratory phase of manual hyperinflation. The oscillations in flow produced may assist in the mobilization of secretions (MacLean *et al.* 1989).
- Tactile stimulation from the physiotherapist's hands, and/or pressure applied before inspiration may produce an increased inspiratory effort (Sumi 1963, Eklund *et al.* 1964).

Positioning and use

- In the treatment of babies and infants, shaking can be applied using two or three fingers against the thorax.
- During self-treatment, many patients practise self-compression during huffing or coughing.

- Compression is often useful in the treatment of the postoperative patient to support an incision during coughing or huffing.

Contraindications
- Manual techniques should not be considered in the presence of frank hemoptysis, over unstable fractures or severe osteoporosis.

Related topics

Impaired gaseous exchange (p. 44); Impaired tracheobronchial clearance (p. 48).

References and further reading

Braun S., Giovannoni R. and O'Connor M. (1984) Improving the cough in patients with spinal cord injury. *Am J Phys Med* **63**: 1–10.

Ekland G., Von Euler C. and Ruteowski S. (1964) Spontaneous and reflex activity of intercostal gamma motorneurones. *J Physiol* **171**: 139–163.

MacClean D., Drummond G., MacPherson C. *et al.* (1989) Maximum expiratory airflow during chest physiotherapy on ventilated patients before and after the application of an abdominal binder. *Intensive Care Medicine* **15**: 396–399.

Sumi T. (1963) The segmental reflex relations of cutaneous afferent inflow to thoracic respiratory motorneurones. *J Neurophysiol* **26**: 478–493.

MECHANICAL VENTILATION (MV)

Description

The provision of a minute volume by external forces. This section will only consider invasive positive pressure ventilation.

Key physiological principles

MV works by:

- supporting/manipulating gas exchange by alveolar ventilation and oxygenation;
- increasing lung volume by augmenting FRC;
- reducing work of breathing by unloading the ventilatory muscles.

The main physiological difference between MV and spontaneous respiration is that during spontaneous respiration a subatmospheric pressure is generated during inspiration, which entrains air into the lungs, whereas, with MV this is replaced by a positive pressure forcing gas into the lungs.

Changes within the respiratory system during MV

- Inspired gas is preferentially distributed to *non-dependent* lung regions causing a ventilation–perfusion mismatch (c.f. positioning to maximize V/Q).
- The combination of position and reduced/absent diaphragmatic action causes a reduction in FRC and therefore lung compliance (c.f. reduced lung volumes, altered respiratory compliance).
- If FRC falls below the closing capacity, atelectasis will occur.
- Surfactant may be adversely affected, further destabilizing airways.
- An artificial airway increases airway resistance.
- Uncontrolled mechanical stress related to pressure, volume and FiO_2 may cause ventilator-acquired lung injury (VALI).
- Mucociliary clearance is impaired.
- The risk of nosocomial pneumonia is increased.
- Altered stimulation of central and peripheral receptors may produce unexpected apneas, dyssynchrony and changes in ventilatory demand (c.f. control of breathing).
- 'Resting' the respiratory muscles may result in atrophy.

Changes within the cardiovascular system during MV

- The raised intrathoracic pressure associated with mechanical ventilation reduces venous return by decreasing the transthoracic pressure gradient (i.e. reduced force 'sucking' blood back to the heart).
- Cardiac output falls as a direct effect of impaired venous return. Consequently, a lower systemic blood pressure may be seen.
- Consequently vital organ perfusion is reduced. Of particular relevance are the brain (increased intracranial pressure), liver (impaired drug clearance, clotting

derangements), gastrointestinal tract (mucosal ulceration) and kidneys (fluid and electrolyte disturbances).
- These effects are further exacerbated in the presence PEEP.
- Hormonal changes (antidiuretic hormone and the renin–angiotensin–aldosterone systems) may predispose to fluid retention.
(Robb 1997a, 1997b)

Clinical relevance

- The diverse physiological effects of mechanical ventilation necessitate multi-system assessment before, during and after treatment. This ensures adequacy of ventilation and cardiovascular/neurological stability, in addition to identifying problems amenable to physiotherapy.
- An 'unstable' patient who requires physiotherapy treatment must be optimized prior to any intervention.
- By understanding and anticipating these physiological effects, physiotherapy treatment can be applied safely and effectively.

Administration

- With conventional MV the patient–ventilator interface may be provided by a cuffed endotracheal tube (oral or nasal), or a cuffed tracheostomy tube.
- Non-invasive ventilation can be provided via a full facemask, nasal mask or mouthpiece (c.f. NIPPV).

Indications for use

- Indications for ventilation include: respiratory rate >30/minute, elevated $PaCO_2$ with pH <7.2 kPa, hypoxemia (P_aO_2:F_iO_2 <27.5), exhaustion, confusion, severe shock, severe LVF, raised intracranial pressure (Singer & Webb 1997).

Monitoring

- Regular arterial blood gas analysis should be performed in order that ventilatory parameters (e.g. rate, tidal volume, FiO_2, PEEP, inspiration/expiration ratio) may be adjusted accordingly.

Modes of ventilation and adjuncts

- Volume-controlled ventilation delivers a pre-set tidal volume, e.g. controlled mandatory ventilation (CMV) and synchronized intermittent mandatory ventilation (SIMV).
- By delivering a set volume the risk of hypoventilation is reduced. However, if respiratory compliance should fall, high airway pressures may be generated. However, modern ventilators limit this danger by offering the option to limit pressure.
- In CMV mode, a predetermined tidal volume is delivered at a preset mandatory respiratory frequency. This mode is generally used with patients who are sedated and/or paralysed.

- In SIMV mode, the ventilator recognizes any patient effort so that a mandatory breath is not superimposed upon the spontaneous breath.
- Pressure-controlled ventilation delivers a preset inspiratory pressure.
- Bi-phasic positive airway pressure (BiPAP) is a form of pressure-controlled ventilation. Pressure alternates between two levels: inspiratory positive airway pressure (IPAP) and expiratory positive airway pressure (EPAP). The difference between the two produces the tidal volume. In this mode spontaneous breathing is possible at any time during the respiratory cycle (Hörmann *et al.* 1994).
- An advantage of pressure-controlled ventilation is a reduced risk of VALI as respiratory compliance is taken into consideration. In addition, it is reported that patient comfort is greater compared to volume-controlled modalities.
- However, hypoventilation is a potential risk if compliance falls dramatically.
- Positive end expiratory pressure (PEEP) describes the positive pressure maintained at the end of expiration during mandatory ventilation. It is recommended that the lowest therapeutic level be used, usually 5–15 cmH_2O.
- Therapeutic effects include: avoidance of end expiratory alveolar collapse, possible alveolar recruitment, increased FRC, improved oxygenation and reduced work of breathing (c.f. reduced lung volumes, altered respiratory compliance).
- CPAP is a spontaneous mode, which provides a positive pressure throughout the respiratory cycle, i.e. inspiration and expiration. As an expiratory pressure is maintained, CPAP provides the beneficial effects of PEEP (c.f. CPAP).
- CPAP is often used as a weaning mode.
- Pressure support ventilation (PSV) is the application of positive pressure to spontaneous breaths. This adjunct reduces the work associated with inspiration, and helps overcome the resistance of tubes and circuitry. Some ventilators offer 'proportional assist' whereby the patient's inspiratory effort is monitored and a suitable level of assistance is provided.

Ventilatory strategies

- Special ventilatory strategies may be implemented in an effort to reduce ventilator-induced lung injury in acute respiratory distress syndrome (Gillette & Hess 2001). These include 'baby lung' approach, permissive hypercapnia (small volumes to prevent VALI), recruitment ventilation (PEEP set at the lower inflection point of the pressure–volume curve to reduce alveolar collapse), and inverse ratio ventilation (inspiratory time ≥50% total respiratory time to address non-compliant lung units with longer filling times).
- Nitric oxide is a potent-inhaled vasodilator, which may be administered to the ventilated patient to reduce ventilation–perfusion defects in severe, acute lung injury.

Precautions

- Patients requiring high levels of PEEP should not be disconnected from the ventilator as alveolar 'de-recruitment' occurs. Repeated alveolar inflation–deflation promotes shear stress and perpetuates lung injury. Similarly loss of therapies such as nitric oxide or inverse ratio ventilation often results in marked patient deterioration.

- The patient–ventilator interface must be handled with care to prevent displacement or damage.

Weaning

- Weaning is defined as the gradual, staged reduction in ventilatory support and its replacement with spontaneous ventilation. CPAP and PSV are commonly used with or without back-up mandatory breaths. NIPPV may be a useful adjunct to the weaning process (c.f. NIPPV).
- Spontaneous breathing should be encouraged and optimized to minimize the adverse physiological effects associated with positive pressure ventilation and promote weaning.
- Factors predicting weaning success include frequency/tidal volume <100 s^{-1} l^{-1} on disconnection, and PaO_2/FiO_2 >27.5 kPa with PEEP <5 cmH_2O (Intensive Care Society National Guidelines 2000).
- Factors preventing weaning are related to excessive respiratory load, inadequate respiratory drive and impaired respiratory pump capacity (c.f. respiratory muscle dysfunction). Physiotherapy intervention is indicated to address specific problems and contribute to the weaning process (Bruton *et al.* 1999).
- Extubation should only be considered when the patient is able to protect the airway, and can cough and swallow effectively.

Related topics

Altered respiratory compliance (p. 23); NIPPV (p. 118); Reduced lung volumes (p. 61); Respiratory failure (p. 63); Respiratory muscle dysfunction (p. 66).

References and further reading

Bruton A., Conway J.H. and Holgate S.T. (1999) Weaning adults from mechanical ventilation: Current issues. *Physiotherapy* **85**(12): 652–661.

Gillette M.A. and Hess D.R. (2001) Ventilator-induced lung injury and the evolution of lung-protective strategies in acute respiratory distress syndrome. *Respir Care* **46**(2): 130–138.

Hörmann C.H., Baum M., Putenson C.H., Mutz N.J. and Benzer H. (1994) Biphasic positive airway pressure (BIPAP) – a new mode of ventilatory support. *Euro J Anaesthesiol* **11**: 37–42.

Intensive Care Society (2000) National Guidelines – when and how to wean. *J Intensive Care Soc* **1**(2).

Robb J. (1997a) Physiological changes occurring with positive pressure ventilation: Part one. *Intens Crit Care Nurs* **13**: 293–307.

Robb J. (1997b) Physiological changes occurring with positive pressure ventilation: Part two. *Intens Crit Care Nurs* **13**: 357–364.

Singer M. and Webb A. (1997) *Oxford Handbook of Critical Care*. Oxford University Press, Oxford.

Tobin M.J. (2001) Advances in mechanical ventilation. *NEJM* **344**(26): 1986–1996.

MOBILIZATION

Description

Mobilization refers to the ability to move, either as a whole or part of the individual. Movement may be brought about actively by the patient, be performed passively by a clinician or result from a combination of both.

Key physiological principles

- Early passive or active mobilization stimulates the musculoskeletal, cardiopulmonary and central nervous systems, limiting the effects of deconditioning.

Clinical relevance

Efficacy

- Short regimes of stretching during a period of immobilization limit adverse connective tissue changes associated with both reduced muscle compliance and range of joint motion. Spinal and thoracic joints should not be overlooked (c.f. thoracic mobilization).
- Active mobilization at an intensity appropriate to the patient's condition may be used to elicit cardiopulmonary and cardiovascular responses to enhance oxygen transport (Dean 1994).
- Early ambulation is an effective method of preventing complications in many low-risk patient groups, e.g. following surgery or uncomplicated MI.
- The combination of exercise and the upright position increases lung volume thereby reducing resistance to flow, improving distribution of gas and facilitating secretion removal (c.f. reduced lung volumes, impaired gaseous exchange, impaired tracheobronchial clearance). Spontaneous cough often occurs with ambulation.

Application

- Passive positioning, movement and stretching are usually achievable with most patients.
- Treatment should be adapted to prevent obstruction of cannulae, to limit discomfort, to comply with orthopedic or surgical requirements and to work within physiological parameters.
- By devising a mobility plan with nursing staff, treatment can be continued with sheet and dressing changes, etc.
- Splinting may be necessary to maintain or regain functional joint position. Neither splinting nor passive exercise should be a substitute for those patients able to perform a full active range of motion.
- In the presence of abnormal muscular tone related to central nervous system pathology, handling and positioning must be modified in order to reduce or increase tone appropriately.

- Mobilization imposes demand upon the cardiopulmonary system. Patients with high levels of cardiopulmonary support may not possess the physiological reserve to meet such additional demands (c.f. mechanical ventilation). Even passive positioning may dramatically increase oxygen consumption in a critically ill patient (Horiuchi *et al.* 1997).
- Individual patient assessment is imperative to avoid an adverse response to mobilization (c.f. assessment).
- The principles of manual exercise therapy and exercise training are adopted, in order that a training response is elicited without causing excessive distress or deterioration (c.f. exercise training).
- Mechanical ventilation in itself does not prevent patient mobilization provided that the interface is protected.
- The physiotherapist should teach patients efficient bed mobility as soon as possible in order to maximize patient independence.
- Safe transfers from bed to chair should be initiated at the earliest opportunity.
- In all patients who have been confined to bed, particularly those with loss of sympathetic dominance or impaired cardiovascular control, hypotension may occur. Therefore, it is vital that progressive sitting occurs for these patients, i.e. gradual assumption of a head-up position.
- Local protocols (e.g. risk assessment, moving and handling, pressure area relief, management of spinal injury patients) should be adhered to.
- Some modern bed frames are designed to facilitate positioning and mobilization. The therapist should be acquainted with all beds in use to ensure optimal use. Low air loss beds may have to be 'firmed' in order to perform passive/active exercises effectively.
- Appropriate seating must be selected prior to patient transfer.
- During ambulation, the therapist may have to contend with lines, drains, catheters, etc. Portable oxygen and a suitable walking aid may be indicated.

Related topics

Deconditioning (p. 32); Effects of general anesthesia (p. 39); Exercise training – 1, 2, 3 & 4 (p. 79); Impaired tracheobronchial clearance (p. 48); Reduced lung volume (p. 61).

References and further reading

Dean E. (1994) Oxygen transport: A physiologically-based conceptual framework for the practice of cardiopulmonary physiotherapy. *Physiotherapy* **80**(6): 347–355.
Horiuchi K., Jordan D., Cohen D., Kemper M.C. and Weissman C. (1997) Insights into the increased oxygen demand during chest physiotherapy. *Crit Care Med* **25**(8): 1347–1351.

NEUROPHYSIOLOGICAL FACILITATION OF RESPIRATION (NPF)

Description

NPF comprises of a set of treatment techniques specifically developed for the respiratory care of the neurologically impaired, self-ventilating adult. NPF techniques have also been used in the neurologically intact adult, however the effects are less pronounced (Bethune 1975).

Six techniques are described:

- co-contraction of the abdomen;
- vertebral pressure of the upper and lower thoracic vertebrae;
- intercostal stretch;
- anterior stretch/posterior basal lift;
- perioral stimulation;
- maintained manual pressure.

Key physiological principles

- Each technique is based upon a different physiological rationale. However, all the techniques are painless, externally applied manual stimuli.
- These provide proprioceptive and tactile stimulation to the patient's mouth, thorax or abdomen.
- The techniques have been proposed to produce reflex involuntary respiratory movements by the patient, which require no conscious co-operation (Bethune 1975).

Clinical relevance

Technique and proposed effect

- Co-contraction of the abdomen. Increases abdominal muscle tone, producing spontaneous coughing in presence of retained secretions. The effects are thought to be produced as a result of muscle spindle activation. Increased abdominal pressure may also cause lower intercostal afferents to fire, increasing diaphragmatic activity (Rood 1973).
- Thoracic vertebral pressure. Increased thoracic and abdominal excursion, facilitating a greater tidal volume. Segmental proprioceptive control of respiration may provide an explanation for the mechanism of this technique. Stimulation of proprioceptors in the lower intercostal and spinal muscles may have reflex control of phrenic motor neurons (Newsome Davis 1970).
- Intercostal stretch. Increased respiratory excursion in area under stretch. Widening the intercostal space stretches the associated muscle. Reflex neuronal activity secondary to muscle spindle activation enhances subsequent respiratory muscle contraction (Eklund *et al.* 1964).

- Anterior stretch/basal lift. Facilitates 'bucket and pump handle' excursion of the ribs. Excitatory skin fields on the thorax produce reflex inspiratory activity. These areas may be recruited by direct cutaneous stimulation (Sumi 1963). Sumi believed that the excitatory skin fields for inspiratory motor neurons were more extensive than those for expiratory neurons, suggesting that a single skin stimulus can cause inspiration. Muscle spindle activation may also occur with this technique.
- Peri-oral stimulation. Increases respiratory excursion and raises level of consciousness. Peri-oral stimulation may elicit a primitive reflex response, which controls respiration and eating in infants. During feeding, the sucking center takes precedence lowering the diaphragm for 5 or more seconds before resuming respiration at a different rhythm (Peiper 1963). Experimentally, peri-oral stimulation has been shown to produce a positive effect on breathing in both neurologically impaired patients and normal individuals (Jones 1997). Rood (1973) suggested that peri-oral stimulation may also reduce spastic muscle tone, however the underlying mechanism is unclear.
- Maintained manual pressure. Increased respiratory excursion in area under contact. Maintained manual contact on the thorax produces cutaneous stimulation, which may provoke reflex intercostal activity (Sumi 1963).

Efficacy

- Anecdotal reports from physiotherapists worldwide using NPF techniques on a variety of patients, describe a 'normalization' of respiratory pattern retained after treatment ceases, a return of mechanical stability of the thorax, and an apparent increase in level of consciousness (Jones 1997). A proven explanatory physiological mechanism is not clear.
- Few scientific studies exist to validate effectiveness. However, on the strength of these positive clinical reports, NPF should still be considered when selecting treatment.
- There is a considerable need for more scientific, supportive evidence.

Indications for use

- NPF techniques are reported to be of use in the treatment of neurologically impaired adult patients who are hypoventilating or have retained secretions (c.f. impaired tracheobronchial clearance, reduced lung volumes).
- NPF techniques may be employed as a first-line treatment for neurologically impaired adults with retained secretions. Abdominal pressure performed by the physiotherapist may assist effective clearance of secretions during spontaneous coughing.
- NPF techniques can also be used to alter respiratory pattern and relieve the symptoms of hyperventilation syndrome (c.f. control of breathing).

Cautions and contraindications

- NPF techniques should not be used to treat children under the age of 7 years because of differences in the anatomy, physiology and neurology of respiration (Bethune 1991).

- NPF techniques should be selected with caution when treating patients with hyperinflated lungs. Bethune (1991) recommends that techniques used to facilitate the intercostal muscles should be avoided as hyperinflation may be exacerbated.

Related topics

Control of breathing (p. 29); Impaired gaseous exchange (p. 44); Impaired tracheobronchial clearance (p. 48); Reduced lung volume (p. 61).

References

Bethune D. (1975) Neurophysiological facilitation of respiration in the unconscious adult patient. *Physiotherapy Canada* 27: 241–245.

Bethune D. (1991) Neurophysiological facilitation of respiration. In: Pryor J.A. (Ed) *Respiratory Care.* Churchill Livingstone, Edinburgh.

Eklund G., von Euler C. and Rutkowski S. (1964) Spontaneous and reflex activity of intercostal gamma motorneurones. *J Physiol* 171: 139–163.

Jones M. (1997) *Neurophysiological Facilitation of Respiration: What Are the Effects?* MSc Physiology, University College, London.

Newsome Davis J. (1970) Spinal control. In: Campbell E.M.J., Agostoni E. and Newsome Davis J. (eds) *The Respiratory Muscle Mechanics and Neural Control.* Saunders, Philadelphia.

Peiper A. (1963) *Cerebral Function in Infancy and Childhood.* Consultants Bureau, New York.

Rood M. (1973) Unpublished lectures given at the University of Western Ontario, London, Ontario.

Sumi T. (1963) The segmental reflex relations of cutaneous afferent inflow to thoracic respiratory motorneurones. *J Neurophysiol* 26: 478–493.

NON-INVASIVE POSITIVE PRESSURE VENTILATION (NIPPV)

Description

A non-invasive form of mechanical ventilation where pressure is applied externally at the nose/mouth (positive pressure device).

N.B. Negative pressure devices such as the Cuirass Jacket or Iron Lung are relatively inefficient especially when impedance to inflation is high. Consequently, positive pressure ventilation is usually the mode of choice. This section will only discuss positive pressure ventilation.

Key physiological principles

- The physiological principles are predominantly the same as for conventional mechanical ventilation:
  - reducing inspiratory muscle work;
  - delivering adequate ventilation;
  - manipulating arterial blood gases.
- However, non-invasive techniques avoid the morbidity and mortality associated with use of artificial airways.

Clinical relevance

Efficacy

NIPPV has been associated with:

- avoidance of intubation or re-intubation;
- improved gas exchange;
- increased exercise capacity;
- reduced work of breathing and sensation of dyspnea;
- prevention of large rises in nocturnal P_aCO_2;
- improved sleep quality;
- increased survival;
- avoidance of tracheostomy;
- improved quality of life
    (Simonds 1996, Abou-Shala & Meduri 1996);
- these benefits are related to many specific patient groups and as such cannot be generalized.

Indications for use

NIPPV may be a hospital- or domiciliary-based service. Indications for use may include:

- Chronic respiratory failure, e.g. neuromuscular disease/injury, chest wall deformity, upper airway disease, intrinsic lung disease, central disorders, particularly for nocturnal support (Simonds & Elliott 1995, Baydur et al. 2000) (c.f. respiratory muscle dysfunction, chest wall deformity/disruption).

- Acute respiratory failure, e.g. postoperative respiratory failure, cardiogenic pulmonary edema, pneumonia, acute exacerbations of CAL (Abou-Shala & Meduri 1996, Plant *et al.* 2000) (c.f. respiratory failure, cardiac failure).
- As a 'bridge' to heart-lung transplantation in those awaiting a donor.
- Weaning from mechanical ventilation (c.f. mechanical ventilation).

Equipment

- Volume-cycled flow generators (e.g. Brompton Pac, PLV Lifecare, Breas) deliver a fixed tidal volume with variable inflation pressure. Breaths may be triggered or imposed depending upon the presence and sufficiency of patients' spontaneous breaths. Useful for patients with very poor chest wall compliance.
- Pressure-cycled flow generators (e.g. Sullivan VPAP, BiPAP, NIPPY) deliver a predetermined airway pressure therefore variable tidal volume. These generators effectively supply pressure support ventilation, which will usually cycle into inspiration in the event of apnea. Variable-flow generators compensate for any leaks at the patient interface. Generally, as effective as volume-cycled flow generators, and better tolerated by patients.
- Bi-level devices allow manipulation of both inspiratory and expiratory positive airway pressure (IPAP and EPAP respectively). EPAP may be used to maintain upper airway patency, improve end expiratory lung volumes, or overcome intrinsic PEEP in lung disease. As the IPAP–EPAP difference is widened, the tidal volume will increase.
- Bi-level therapy effectively combines the effects of IPPB or inspiratory pressure support and CPAP (Denehy & Berney 2001).
- Oxygen, humidification and nebulized drugs may be administered during NIPPV (pre-set volume or pressure) (c.f. oxygen therapy and humidification).
- General-purpose intensive care ventilators can be used for NIPPV, provided that they can accommodate for leaks.

Administration

- Clear nasal or full-face masks are the most commonly used patient–ventilator interfaces. Occasionally, mouthpieces or nasal pillows are used.
- Nasal masks are more comfortable, have a lower dead space, and allow speech, expectoration and mouth care.
- If necessary, nasal masks can be used with a chin strap to control leaks.
- Granuflex™ dressing over the bridge of the nose reduces the incidence of ulceration.
- Accurate interface selection is essential to NIPPV success.

Contraindications and precautions

- NIPPV may not be appropriate when the patient is unco-operative or agitated.
- NIPPV is contraindicated if the patient is unable to protect their airway or clear secretions.
- Patients presenting with overt respiratory failure and requiring urgent intubation are unsuitable candidates for NIPPV.
- Disorders of other systems may preclude NIPPV, e.g. impending multiorgan failure, extreme metabolic acidosis, hemodynamic insufficiency, paralytic ileus.

- An inadequate seal at the patient–ventilator interface may render NIPPV impossible.
- NIPPV may cause nasal pressure sores, painful eyes and abdominal distention when applied injudiciously or with inadequate monitoring.
- Leaks during inspiration will result in less effective ventilation.
- Upper airway obstruction may occur if the cycling pressure falls below the closing pressure of the upper airway.

Recommendations

- Settings should be adjusted to match the patient's respiratory pattern – starting with a small tidal volume using a volume-controlled machine, or relatively low inspiratory/expiratory positive airway pressures with a pressure-controlled machine.
- Trial breaths allow the patient to become accustomed to the mask and gas flow, and permit the clinician to adjust the settings to match the patient's respiratory pattern.
- The clinician should ensure that the patient knows how to disconnect the tubing from the mask in case of emergency.
- Monitoring is essential for safe and effective NIPPV. Recommended measurements include pulse oximetry, capnography, ABGs, pressure alarms, exhaled tidal volumes and chest wall movement to ensure synchronization between patient and ventilator.
- Improvement in arterial blood gases within 1 hour of NIPPV instigation may be a predictor of successful intervention (Abou-Shala & Meduri 1996) (c.f. assessment).
- The physiotherapist may choose a bi-level device as an alternative to IPPB or CPAP in the treatment of refractory respiratory complications. To date, there is no comparative research to evaluate this practice (Denehy & Berney 2001).
- Successful instigation of NIPPV may allow effective airway clearance treatment in a patient who was previously too breathless or fatigued.

Related topics

CPAP (p. 76); IPPB (p. 99); Mechanical ventilation (p. 109); Respiratory failure (p. 63).

References and further reading

Abou-Shala N. and Meduri U. (1996) Non-invasive mechanical ventilation in patients with acute respiratory failure. *Crit Care Med* 24(4): 705–715.

Antonelli M. and Conti G. (2000) Non-invasive positive pressure ventilation as treatment for acute respiratory failure in critically ill patients. *Crit Care* 4(1): 15–22.

Baydur A., Layne E., Aral H., Krishnareddy T., Topacio R., Frederick G. and Bodden W. (2000) Long term non-invasive ventilation in the community for patients with musculoskeletal disorders: 46 years experience and review. *Thorax* 55(1): 4–11.

Denehy L. and Berney S. (2001) The use of positive pressure devices by physiotherapists. *Eur Respir J* 17: 821–829.

Plant P.K., Owen J.L. and Elliott M.W. (2000) Early use of non-invasive ventilation for acute exacerbations of chronic obstructive pulmonary disease on general respiratory wards: a multicentre randomised controlled trial. *Lancet* 355: 1931–1935.

Simonds A. (ed) (1996) *Non-invasive Respiratory Support*. Chapman and Hall, London.

Simonds A.K. and Elliott M.W. (1995) Outcome of domiciliary NIPPV in restrictive and obstructive disorders. *Thorax* 50(6): 595–596.

OXYGEN THERAPY

Description

Oxygen therapy is a drug regime, which may be delivered with a variety of devices and concentrations.

Key physiological principles

- Used therapeutically to increase alveolar oxygen tension, by increasing the oxygen concentration in the inspired gas above 0.21.
- Oxygen therapy increases oxygen transport by insuring that hemoglobin is fully saturated and raising the quantity of oxygen in solution in the plasma. The work of breathing required to maintain a specific arterial oxygen tension is therefore reduced (Bateman & Leach 1998).

Clinical relevance

Efficacy

- Long-term oxygen therapy (LTOT) has been associated with improved exercise capacity, reduced dyspnea, reduced pulmonary hypertension, improved quality of life and a decrease in nocturnal hypoxemia in patients with CAL (Barnes 1999).
- Supplemental peri-operative oxygen therapy reduces the incidence of surgical wound infection (Greif *et al.* 2000).

Indications for use

- The absolute indication for oxygen therapy is hypoxemia (<7.8 kPa).
- Instances where oxygen therapy may be used empirically include: cardiac/respiratory arrest, myocardial infarction with associated hypoxemia, shock, postoperatively, hypotension (systolic BP <100 mmHg), increased metabolic demands, e.g. major burns or trauma, carbon monoxide poisoning, or anticipated hypoxemia, e.g. during tracheal suction.
- The British Thoracic Society CAL Guidelines (1997) recommend prescription of LTOT if the P_aO_2 is <7.3 kPa.

Administration

- Oxygen should be prescribed on the drug/anesthetic chart or in the medical notes.
- Prescription should cover flow rate, delivery system, duration and monitoring (Bateman & Leach 1998).
- When O_2 is administered by mask at flow rates >4 l/min, or delivered directly to the trachea, supplemental humidification is recommended (Bateman & Leach 1998) (c.f. humidification).

- Oxygen therapy is discontinued when arterial oxygenation is adequate with the patient breathing room air and vital signs are consistent with resolution of tissue hypoxia (Bateman & Leach 1998) (c.f. impaired gaseous exchange).

Fixed performance devices e.g. Venturi valves
- The device delivers premixed gas at a flow rate greater than the patient's inspiratory flow rate. As such, the device can provide the entire inspirate.
- The venturi system creates a 'Bernoulli' effect whereby an accurate, large volume of room air is entrained by the device as oxygen flows over the valve. The ratio of oxygen to entrained air is fixed and accurate (24–60%).
- As the device entrains room air, adequate humidification of the inspired gas will take place.
- Humidification devices should not be used in conjunction with a separate venturi valve as water droplets condense in the valve outlets altering the F_iO_2 delivered. N.B. Some specific humidification devices work on a venturi system – these are safe to use.
- Fixed-performance devices are appropriate for patients with variable patterns of breathing, or for those who require an accurate FiO_2. The high flow rates minimize re-breathing.

Variable performance devices e.g. nasal cannulae, Hudson face masks
- The device provides only part of the inspirate, the patient must also breathe in room air to achieve an adequate minute volume. Consequently the ratio of oxygen (delivered by the device) to air (entrained from the room) is variable.
- The FiO_2 is dependent upon minute volume and oxygen flow rate.
- Nasal cannulae should not be used with a flow rate >4 l/min because of the risk of nasal mucosal irritation. Consequently humidification should never be required.
- Variable-flow devices are suitable for patients with an adequate respiratory rate and regular pattern of breathing, where hypoxemia and hypercapnia are not a major concern.

Reservoir device e.g. Trauma mask
- A large-capacity, variable-performance device. The patient breathes from a reservoir of oxygen below the mask. A valve system ensures that the majority of gas inhaled is from the reservoir and that breath is exhaled mainly via ports in the mask.
- The system can achieve a FiO_2 of >60%, however rebreathing may occur because of the low flow rate. The flow meter should be set such that the reservoir bag remains inflated during inspiration.

Monitoring
- Monitoring is imperative in order to detect and respond to any adverse effects.
- Noninvasive pulse oximetry and/or arterial blood gas analysis allows appropriate titration of the FiO_2. If arterial blood gases are available, the $P_aO_2:F_iO_2$ ratio may be calculated (e.g. 13 kPa/0.21 = 62).

- Pulse oximetry alone may mask inadequate gas exchange and progressive hypercapnia.
- The flow meter and delivery device should be regularly checked for accuracy and patency. An oxygen analyzer may be used within the delivery system to ensure an accurate F_iO_2.
- The patient should be assessed subjectively, e.g. dyspnea and comfort, during oxygen therapy.

Dangers

- An inappropriate concentration of oxygen may have serious or lethal effects.
- Long-term CAL patients who retain CO_2 may develop hypercapnia as a result of oxygen administration. This is because these patients rely on a central hypoxic drive to breathe, which is inhibited with supplemental O_2 therapy. This leads to hypoventilation and/or the reversal of hypoxic pulmonary vasoconstriction causing V/Q mismatching (Crossley *et al.* 1997) (c.f. impaired gaseous exchange).
- Pulmonary O_2 toxicity has been demonstrated experimentally. Effects may include increased permeability and cytological change within the pulmonary capillary bed endothelium and thickening of the alveolar/capillary membrane. It is advisable to minimize the F_iO_2 when possible.
- High concentrations of oxygen can displace inert nitrogen within the lung. The loss of this 'cushion' may result in small areas of collapse (absorption atelectasis) in areas of lung with low ventilation/perfusion ratios (c.f. reduced lung volumes). This is of particular significance for patients who are unable to deep breathe effectively.
- Oxygen is a combustible gas.
- The clinician should address issues of patient discomfort, e.g. appropriate device selection, adequate humidification. Dependency upon oxygen therapy should be discouraged.
- Eye damage (retrolental fibroplasia) has been attributed to hyperoxia in neonates.

Related topics

Derangements in acid–base balance (p. 17); Effects of general anesthesia (p. 39); Humidification (p. 94); Impaired gaseous exchange (p. 44); Respiratory failure (p. 63); Ventilation/perfusion mismatch (p. 136).

References and further reading

Barnes P.J. (1999) *Managing Chronic Obstructive Pulmonary Disease.* Science Press Ltd., London.
Bateman N.T. and Leach R.M. (1998) ABC of oxygen: Acute oxygen therapy. *BMJ* **317** (7161): 798–801.
BTS guidelines for the management of chronic obstructive pulmonary disease: The COPD Guideline Group of the Standards of Care Committee of the BTS (1997). *Thorax* **52**(suppl 5): S1–S28.

Crossley D.J., McGuire G.P., Barrow P.M. and Houston P.L. (1997) Influence of inspired oxygen concentration on dead space, respiratory drive and PaCO$_2$ in intubated patients with COPD. *Crit Care Med* 25 (9): 1522–1552.

Greif R., Akca O., Horn E.P., Kurz A. and Sessler D.I. (2000) Supplemental perioperative oxygen to reduce the incidence of surgical wound infection. *NEJM* 342(3): 161–167.

PHYSIOTHERAPY MANAGEMENT OF PAIN

Description

This section is intended to provide an overview of modalities, which may be used when treating patients with co-existing cardiopulmonary dysfunction, e.g. a postoperative patient, a trauma patient on ICU or a CAL out-patient with musculoskeletal dysfunction.

Key physiological principles

Physiotherapy treatment modalities may intervene in the transmission of nociceptive input at a number of key stages:

- Peripheral level (e.g. removal of chemical irritants and alteration of cell permeability).
- Spinal segmental level (e.g. segmental inhibition and physiological blocking mechanisms).
- Supraspinal level (e.g. descending inhibitory control mechanisms and diffuse noxious inhibitory control).
- Cortical level (e.g. placebo effect, cognitive strategies and behavior modification)
  (Walsh 1991, Melzack & Wall 1996).

Consequently, thorough assessment and appropriate technique selection are essential both to assess the origin of the pain, and activate the required pain-suppressing mechanism (Walsh 1991).

Modalities: indications and efficacy

Transcutaneous electrical nerve stimulation (TENS)
- TENS is believed to work at a spinal segmental level via the pain gate theory. In addition, it acts at a supraspinal level by stimulating descending inhibitory control systems (Melzack & Wall 1996).
- Variable modes may be used, e.g. high frequency, low intensity (acute pain), or low frequency, high intensity (chronic pain).
- Although TENS has been advocated in the treatment of postoperative pain, musculoskeletal pain and neurogenic pain (Grady & Severn 1997), some studies have shown conflicting results suggestive of a placebo effect (Domaille & Reeves 1997).

Acupuncture
- Many theories have been suggested to explain the analgesic effects of Western Approach Acupuncture. These include neurological mechanisms (e.g. pain gate theory, descending inhibitory control systems, viscero-somatic reflexes, diffuse noxious inhibitory control), neurohumoral mechanisms (e.g. endorphin release, modulation of neurotransmitters) and psychological mechanisms (e.g. the placebo effect) (Lewith & Kenyon 1984).

- Although, acupuncture is classically considered a treatment for acute and chronic pain, interest is increasing regarding the effects of acupuncture on respiratory conditions.

Heat therapy
- Tissue may be heated superficially via heated packs, or deeply via ultrasound or electromagnetic radiation.
- The analgesic effects are thought to be mediated via vasodilation of superficial and deep blood vessels (removing nociceptive agents and augmenting delivery of cells/chemicals necessary for healing), and at a spinal segmental level (closing the pain gate) (Melzack & Wall 1996).
- Hydrotherapy combines superficial warmth and buoyancy and is often used for patients presenting with neuromuscular problems. However, in patients with lung disease, the effect of immersion on vital capacity may be detrimental (Anstey & Roskell 2000).

Cold therapy
- Cold therapy is a form of hyperstimulation analgesia. The intense sensory input may activate diffuse noxious inhibitory controls, similar to that postulated for acupuncture.
- In addition to its analgesic properties, cold therapy has experimentally shown a decrease in inflammatory reaction. Consequently, it is often used to reduce the recovery time following acute and chronic injuries (Swenson et al. 1996).
- Reflex activity and motor function are impaired following cold therapy, therefore the physiotherapist should be vigilant to ensure further injury does not occur in the subsequent 30 minutes (MacAuley 2001).
- As the physiological effects are dependent upon temperature reduction in the tissues, factors such as method and duration of application are critical. Following a systematic review, repeated ice application of 10 minutes duration is recommended (MacAuley 2001).

Manual therapy (e.g. joint mobilization, soft tissue stretching, massage)
- Much of the theory regarding these modalities is covered in the Thoracic Mobilization chapter.
- These techniques are often employed after injury, surgery or immobility, e.g. painful/reduced glenohumeral and scapulothoracic range of movement post-thoracotomy, or spinal pain following a protracted period of bed rest.
- Neural tissue should also be considered in assessment/treatment (Butler 2000).
- Trigger point stimulation is a therapy that produces descending inhibition over a large area. It is believed to work via descending diffuse noxious inhibitory controls (see acupuncture and cold therapy).

Cognitive strategies
- Cognitive strategies attempt to reduce the sensation of pain via modification of thought processes.
- These techniques include relaxation (e.g. Contrast, Reciprocal and Suggestion Methods) and patient education.
- Encouraging the patient to relax the shoulder girdle, unclench the hands and

jaw, and move the tongue away from the roof of the mouth may facilitate 'Mini-relaxation' sessions.

- Patient education is essential in order that patients understand their pain and appreciate their role in its management, e.g. advice regarding use of patient-controlled analgesia or wound support, and coping strategies (Walsh 1991).

Related topics

Chest wall deformity/dysfunction (p. 26); Deconditioning (p. 32); Pain (p. 58); Thoracic mobilization (p. 143).

References and further reading

Anstey K.H. and Roskell C. (2000) Hydrotherapy: Detrimental or beneficial to the respiratory system? *Physiotherapy* 86(1): 5–13.

Butler S. (2000) *The Sensitive Nervous System*. Noigroup Publications, Adelaide.

Domaille M. and Reeves B. (1997) TENS and pain control after coronary artery bypass surgery. *Physiotherapy* 83(10): 510–516.

Grady K.M. and Severn A.M. (1997) *Key Topics in Chronic Pain*. Bios Scientific Publishers, Oxford.

Lewith G.T. and Kenyon J.N. (1984) Physiological and psychological explanations for the mechanism of acupuncture as a treatment for chronic pain. *Social Science Med* 19: 1367–1378.

MacAuley D.C. (2001) Ice therapy: how good is the evidence? *Int J Sports Med* 22(5): 379–384.

Melzack R. and Wall P.D. (1996) *The Challenge of Pain*, 2nd edition. Penguin Books, London.

Swenson C., Sward L. and Karlsson J. (1996) Cryotherapy in sports medicine. *Scand J Med Sci Sports* 6(4): 193–200.

Walsh D. (1991) Nociceptive pathways – relevance to the physiotherapist. *Physiotherapy* 77(5): 317–321.

POSITIONING 1 – GRAVITY-ASSISTED POSITIONING (GAP)

Description

The specific positioning of a patient, utilizing gravity in order to drain a particular broncho-pulmonary segment. This technique is not used in isolation, but as an adjunct to the active cycle of breathing techniques, and in conjunction with manual techniques.

Key physiological principles

- Each bronchopulmonary segment is a functionally independent unit of lung, supplied by a separate bronchus.
- Appropriate positioning can place the bronchus of each bronchopulmonary segment perpendicular to gravity. This allows gravitational forces to assist the movement of bronchial secretions.

Clinical relevance

Efficacy

- The positions used for GAP are based on the anatomy of the bronchial tree (Nelson 1934) and are accepted by the Thoracic Society (1950).
- GAP can be used to assist the clearance of excess bronchial secretions (Hofmeyr et al. 1986). A thorough assessment will identify the GAP necessary to maximize removal of secretions.
- The exact anatomy of each bronchus supplying a bronchopulmonary segment may vary slightly from patient to patient. Therefore, some modification of position may be necessary to optimize sputum clearance.
- GAP is rarely used in isolation, but as an adjunct to the ACBT (c.f. ACBT).
- Where appropriate, maximum clearance of secretions can be facilitated by the administration of a bronchodilator agent prior to physiotherapy treatment.
- More than one GAP may be required in one treatment session, although thorough treatment of one bronchopulmonary segment should be completed before a second position is used.
- Cecins et al. (1999) concluded that the modified horizontal position was as effective as a head-down position in terms of wet sputum production in bronchiectatic subjects. Furthermore, the sensation of breathlessness during treatment was reduced with the horizontal position, and generally preferred by the patients.
- Continuous lateral rotational therapy using kinetic beds may offer a method of modified GAP in critically ill patients. However, to be effective the angle of rotation must be considered (Dolovich et al. 1998).

Indications for use

- GAP can be used effectively in both children and adults in the treatment of excess sputum production.

- Effective positioning can be gained with babies positioned over the physiotherapist's knee.
- GAP is unlikely to be of benefit in patients with very tenacious secretions.
- GAP can be taught and used as part of a self-treatment regime.
- A variety of portable tables and wedges are commercially available to enable effective GAP to be carried out independently in the home.

Contraindications and cautions

- Positions should be modified to accommodate the breathless patient (c.f. positioning to relieve breathlessness), cardiac failure, cardiovascular instability (c.f. cardiac failure), neurological instability following esophageal surgery unexplained hemoptysis and in infants with esophageal reflux and following esophageal surgery.
- In critically ill patients, positioning may elicit exercise or stress-like responses, resulting in increased oxygen consumption (Horiuchi *et al.* 1997). Evaluation of individual patient response is recommended.
- GAP may have significant effects on ventilation homogeneity that may predispose the patient to arterial desaturation (Ross *et al.* 1992) (c.f. impaired gaseous exchange). Ideally pulse oximetry should be used to safeguard the patient.

Related topics

Impaired gaseous exchange (p. 44); Impaired tracheobronchial clearance (p. 48).

References and further reading

Cecins N.M., Jenkins S.C., Pengelly J. and Ryan G. (1999) The ACBT – to tip or not to tip. *Respir Med* 93(9): 660–665.

Dolovich M., Rushbrook J., Churchill E., Mazza M. and Powles A.C. (1998) Effect of continuous lateral rotational therapy on lung mucus transport in mechanically ventilated patients. *J Crit Care* 13(3): 119–125.

Hofmeyr J.L., Webber B.A. and Hodson M.E. (1986) Evaluation of positive expiratory pressure as an adjunct to chest physiotherapy in the treatment of cystic fibrosis. *Thorax* 41: 951–954.

Horiuchi K., Jordan D., Cohen D., Kemper M.C. and Weissman C. (1997) Insights into the increased oxygen demand during chest physiotherapy. *Crit Care Med* 25(8): 1347–1351.

Houtmeyers E., Gosselink R., Gayan-Ramirez G. and Decramer M. (1999) Regulation of mucociliary clearance in health and disease. *Euro Respir J* 13: 1177–1188.

Nelson H.P. (1934) Postural drainage of the lungs. *BMJ* 2: 251–255.

Ross J., Dean E. and Abboud R.T. (1992) The effect of postural drainage positioning on ventilation homogeneity in healthy subjects. *Phys Ther* 72(11): 794–799.

Thoracic Society (1950) The nomenclature of the bronchopulmonary anatomy. *Thorax* 5: 222–228.

POSITIONING 2 – TO RELIEVE BREATHLESSNESS

Description

The positioning of a patient in order to utilize the therapeutic benefits of specific relaxed positions, used in conjunction with breathing control.

Key physiological principles

- Standing or leaning forward moves the abdominal contents so that the anterior portion of the diaphragm is raised.
- This optimizes the length tension status of the diaphragm and may facilitate diaphragmatic contraction during inspiration (Sharp *et al.* 1980, O'Neill & McCarthy 1983, Dean 1985) that may reduce the work of breathing.
- The same effect may be gained by positioning a patient in side lying or high side lying, where the curvature of the dependent part of the diaphragm is increased facilitating contraction during inspiration.

Clinical relevance

Efficacy

- Often of benefit to the breathless patient, especially when used in conjunction with breathing control (c.f. ACBT).
- Appropriate positioning should incorporate relaxation of the head and jaw, neck and shoulders. This minimizes the use of accessory muscles and encourages the patient to adopt a more efficient breathing pattern.
- Effective positions include high side lying, forward lean sitting, relaxed standing and forward lean standing.

Indications for use

- In some instances an acutely or chronically breathless patient will instinctively adopt a position of ease to relieve breathlessness.
- Assessment of an acutely breathless patient can be performed while the subject is in a relaxed position.
- Relaxed positions can be used instead of GAP during physiotherapy treatment to remove excess bronchial secretions (c.f. GAP). In this instance the emphasis will be on breathing control when using the ACBT.
- These positions can be taught and modified for used at home during an acute exacerbation of breathlessness, whilst stair climbing or when mobilizing over longer distances (c.f. mobilization).

Related topics

Airflow limitation (p. 26); Altered respiratory compliance (p. 23); Control of breathing (p. 29); Deconditioning (p. 32); Reduced lung volume (p. 61).

References and further reading

Dean E. (1985) Effect of body position on pulmonary function. *Physical Therapy* **65**: 613–618.

O'Neil S.O. and McCarthy D.S. (1983) Postural relief of dyspnoea in severe chronic airflow limitation: relationship to respiratory muscle strength. *Thorax* **38**: 595–600.

Sharp J.T., Drutz W.S., Moisan T., Forester J. and Machnach W. (1980) Postural relief of dyspnoea in severe chronic obstructive pulmonary disease. *Am Rev Respir Dis* **122**: 201–211.

POSITIONING 3 – TO IMPROVE LUNG VOLUME

Description

The positioning of a patient in order to improve both lung volume and the distribution of ventilation.

Key physiological principles

- The action of gravity on the lung produces the pleural pressure gradient (West 2000). This pleural pressure gradient influences the normal distribution of ventilation. Consequently, at FRC or above, the dependent lung regions receive a greater proportion of the inspired volume.
- If FRC falls below closing capacity (CC), airway closure occurs during tidal breathing (c.f. reduced lung volumes). Airway closure will occur first in the dependent lung regions.
- In this situation, the non-dependent lung regions become the most compliant and therefore receive a greater proportion of ventilation (c.f. altered respiratory compliance).
- These effects (reduced lung volume and altered distribution of gas) produce a low V/Q relationship (c.f. impaired gaseous exchange) (Hess *et al.* 1992, Tucker & Jenkins 1996).
- In the supine position, the action of gravity upon the rib cage, diaphragm and abdominal contents causes a progressive reduction in FRC compared to erect posture (Jenkins *et al.* 1988).

Clinical relevance

Efficacy

- FRC may be manipulated by postural modification (Jenkins *et al.* 1988).
- In normal subjects FRC is greatest in standing, and is progressively reduced with the following positions:
  - sitting;
  - half lying (backrest at 45° with two pillows for support);
  - left side lying or right side lying;
  - slumped sitting or supine
  (Jenkins et al 1988).
- FRC declines by 14% with a change from sitting to half lying (Jenkins *et al.* 1988). This may be of great consequence in a sick patient.
- Evidence suggests that upright position combined with lower thoracic expansion exercises (LTEE) utilizing low flow rates (c.f. ACBT), improves ventilation to the dependent zones (Tucker & Jenkins 1996).
- It has been proposed that in the side lying position the distribution of ventilation to the non-dependent lung may improve when combined with LTEE. The proposed mechanisms include:

- improved chest wall expansion and compliance;
- respiratory muscle activation;
- a greater negative intrapleural pressure gradient.

However, this method of increasing 'regional ventilation' is unsubstantiated (Tucker & Jenkins 1996).

Indications for use
- Patients with impaired gaseous exchange secondary to a reduction in FRC.
- All major surgical procedures result in a reduction in FRC (c.f. effects of general anesthesia). Consequently, body positioning and early mobilization may be instrumental in addressing this problem.
- Particular attention should be paid to those with an already diminished FRC or elevated CC, e.g. elderly, obese, smokers, airflow limitation (Jenkins *et al.* 1988).

Application
- It is recommended that patients be sat out of bed and/or mobilized as soon as feasibly possible to increase FRC.
- All members of the multiprofessional team should be aware of the adverse effects of slumped sitting. Side lying offers a suitable alternative to sitting if the patient is confined to bed.
- When using LTEE in combination with positioning, greatest effect, in terms of distribution of ventilation, is likely to be achieved with an upright position and a slow inspiratory flow rate.
- Positioning to improve both ventilation and maximize ventilation/perfusion ratio, is likely to be most effective in improving gaseous exchange (Dean 1985) (c.f. positioning to maximize ventilation/perfusion ratio).

Contraindications and cautions
- In critically ill patients, positioning may elicit exercise or stress-like responses, resulting in increased oxygen consumption (Horiuchi *et al.* 1997). Evaluation of individual patient response is recommended.

Related topics

ACBT (p. 71); Altered respiratory compliance (p. 23); Effects of general anesthesia (p. 39); Impaired gaseous exchange (p. 44); Reduced lung volume (p. 61).

References and further reading

Dean E. (1985) Effect of position on pulmonary function. *Physical Therapy* 65(5): 613–618.

Hess D., Agarwal N.N. and Myers C.L. (1992) Positioning, lung function and kinetic bed therapy. *Respiratory Care* 37(2): 181–197.

Horiuchi K., Jordan D., Cohen D., Kemper M.C. and Weissman C. (1997) Insights into the increased oxygen demand during chest physiotherapy. *Crit Care Med* 25(8): 1347–1351.

Jenkins S.C., Soutar S.A. and Moxham J. (1988) The effects of posture on lung volumes in normal subjects and in patients pre and post-coronary artery surgery. *Physiotherapy* 74(10): 492–496.

Tucker B. and Jenkins S. (1996) The effect of breathing exercises with body positioning on regional lung ventilation. *Aust J Physio* **42**(3): 219–227.

West J.B. (2000) *Respiratory Physiology – The Essentials*, 6th edition. Lippencott, Williams & Wilkins, Philadelphia.

POSITIONING 4 – TO MAXIMIZE VENTILATION/PERFUSION RATIO

Description

For gaseous exchange to take place it is necessary to have an adequate perfusion of blood and a regular supply of inspired air. In order to maximize oxygenation, ventilation and perfusion must be optimal in the same areas. In situations of pathology, specific positioning of patients can improve oxygenation by matching ventilation to perfusion.

Key physiological principles

- In the self-ventilating adult, ventilation and perfusion are both preferentially distributed to the dependent areas of the lungs (West 2000).
- In adults receiving positive pressure ventilation, perfusion is still preferentially distributed to the dependent regions of the lungs, however, maximum ventilation occurs in non-dependent regions.
- All lungs have some degree of ventilation/perfusion (V/Q) inequality. In the normal upright lung this occurs in a regional pattern with V/Q ratio decreasing from apex to base.

Clinical relevance

Efficacy

- When areas of lung have a mismatch of ventilation and/or perfusion, gas transfer becomes less efficient. As a result, hypoxia and/or hypercapnia may occur (c.f. impaired gaseous exchange).
- By positioning a patient to maximize V/Q ratio, oxygenation can be optimized.
- An increase in S_aO_2 may be seen within a few minutes of appropriate positioning.

Positioning and indications for use

- Any patient with abnormal ventilation, e.g. atelectasis or consolidation, or abnormal perfusion, e.g. pulmonary embolus, will benefit from specific positioning to maximize V/Q ratio (c.f. disorders of the pulmonary circulation).
- In the self-ventilating adult with unilateral lung disease, gas transfer may be maximized by positioning the patient in side lying with the unaffected lung in a dependent position (Zack 1974).
- In the self-ventilating adult with bilateral disease, assessment skills such as auscultation and CXR analysis should be used to determine which lung or lobes of the lungs are least affected (c.f. assessment). The least-affected lobes should be placed in a dependent position in order to maximize oxygenation.
- In cases where disease is uniform, positioning the patient with the right lung in a dependent position may be advantageous, as it has a slightly larger surface area and is not subject to cardiac compression.

- Positive pressure ventilation in adults will always produce a V/Q mismatch. This is because perfusion increases down the upright lung, whereas the non-dependent lung now becomes preferentially ventilated as a result of changes in respiratory mechanics. In this instance, a regular change in position is recommended, using both left and right lateral plus high sitting, to ensure adequate ventilation of all lung regions (c.f. mechanical ventilation). Kinetic beds may be used which provide continuous lateral rotational therapy (Bein *et al.* 1998).

Contraindications and cautions
- In critically ill patients, positioning may elicit exercise or stress-like responses, resulting in increased oxygen consumption (Horiuchi *et al.* 1997). Evaluation of individual patient response is recommended.

Related topics

Impaired gaseous exchange (p. 44); Reduced lung volumes (p. 61).

References and further reading

Bein T., Reber A., Metz C., Jauch K.W. and Hedenstierna G. (1998) Acute effects of continuous lateral rotational therapy on ventilation perfusion inequality in lung injury. *Intens Care Med* 24(2): 132–137.

Dean E. (1985) Effect of position on pulmonary function. *Phys Ther* 65(5): 613–618.

Horiuchi K., Jordan D., Cohen D., Kemper M.C. and Weissman C. (1997) Insights into the increased oxygen demand during chest physiotherapy. *Crit Care Med* 25(8): 1347–1351.

West J.B. (2000) *Respiratory Physiology – The Essentials*, 6th edition. Lippencott, Williams & Wilkins, Philadelphia.

Zack M.B., Pontoppidan H. and Kazemi H. (1974) The effect of lateral positions on gas exchange in pulmonary disease. *Am Rev Respir Dis* 110: 49–55.

POSITIONING 5 – PRONE POSITIONING

Description

The turning of a patient from supine to the prone position.

Key physiological principles

Several theories have been proposed to explain the benefits gained from prone positioning; increased FRC, re-expansion of gravity-induced atelectasis, re-distribution of perfusion and alteration in diaphragmatic mechanics. However, most interest has been in the effects of prone positioning on V/Q relationships.

- Placing a patient in the prone position may lead to beneficial changes in respiratory mechanics (Pelosi et al. 1998). With positive pressure mechanical ventilation in the supine position (ribs and sternum free to move), preferential ventilation occurs in the nondependent/anterior regions of the lung. In the prone position however, the anterior/sternal portion of the chest wall is 'splinted'. This reduces regional compliance, and effects a more homogenous distribution of ventilation.
- A gravitational gradient of pulmonary perfusion (increasing down the upright lung) is widely accepted (West et al. 1964). Experimental work suggests that this gradient is reduced in the prone position producing a more uniform distribution of perfusion compared to other positions (Hakim et al. 1988). Overall, the net effect of these two factors is an improvement in V/Q matching and therefore oxygenation.

Clinical relevance

Efficacy

- Prone positioning was first proposed over 20 years ago (Piehl & Brown 1976), but has only relatively recently been clinically applied on a wide scale.
- Prone positioning improves oxygenation in approximately 70% of patients with ALI/ARDS (Chatte et al. 1997).
- Although prone positioning may influence physiological values, in clinical trials its use has not been shown to increase survival. However, this may be attributable to several factors; difficulty in identifying those patients likely to benefit from prone positioning, when to instigate this intervention and for how long.
- Currently, patients are left prone for between 6 and 12 hours.
- The successful use of prone positioning often allows for a reduction in PEEP, nitric oxide administration and/or F_iO_2 (c.f. mechanical ventilation, oxygen therapy).

Complications

- Pressure necrosis over bony prominences.
- Nerve compression secondary to poor positioning and muscle wasting.

- Retinal damage secondary to increased intra-occular pressure.
- Swelling to the face/neck due to venous stasis.
- Dislodging intravenous lines or chest drains.
- Risk of dislodging endotracheal/tracheostomy tube.

Contraindications
- Multiple trauma.
- Spinal instability.
- Raised intracranial pressure.
- Shock.
- Acute bleeding.
- Recent abdominal surgery.

Related topics

Altered respiratory compliance (p. 23); Derangements in acid–base balance (p. 17); Infection/inflammation (p. 57); Respiratory failure (p. 63); Ventilation/perfusion mismatch (p. 136).

References and further reading

Chatte G., Sab J., Dubois J., Sirodot M., Gaussorges P. and Robert D. (1997) Prone position in mechanically ventilated patients with severe acute respiratory failure. *Am J Respir Crit Care Med* **155**: 473–478.

Hakim T.S., Dean G.W. and Lisbona R. (1988) Effect of body posture on spatial distribution of pulmonary blood flow. *J Appl Physiol* **64**: 1160–1170.

Pelosi P., Tubiolo D., Mascheroni D., Viscardi P., Crotti S., Valenza F. and Gattinoni L. (1998) Effects of prone positioning on respiratory mechanics and gas exchange during acute lung injury. *Am J Respir Crit Care Med* **157**: 387–393.

Piehl M.A. and Brown R.S. (1976) Use of extreme position changes in respiratory failure. *Crit Care Med* **4**: 13–14.

West J.B., Dollery C.T. and Naimark A. (1964) Distribution of blood flow in isolated lung; relation to vascular and alveolar pressures. *J Appl Physiol* **19**: 713–724.

POSITIVE EXPIRATORY PRESSURE (PEP)

Description

The PEP system either consists of a fitted facemask with a one-way valve, in which expiratory pressure resistors are inserted, or a mouthpiece device with adjustable expiratory resistance. A manometer may be incorporated into the system to assess performance.

Key physiological principles

- The production of PEP increases end-expiratory lung volume, therefore reducing airway resistance and small airway closure (West 2000).
- As a result, channels of collateral ventilation are recruited allowing air to flow behind sputum plugs, thus facilitating secretion movement.

Clinical relevance

Efficacy

- The use of a PEP mask was first described by Falk *et al.* (1984). This group reported an increased quantity of sputum and an increase in transcutaneous oxygen tension, during a comparative trial with 'conventional physiotherapy' (GAP and percussion). Furthermore, PEP was more popular with the patients. It should be noted that GAP and percussion are rarely used in isolation, but as adjuncts to the ACBT (c.f. ACBT, GAP, manual techniques).
- A study by van der Schans (1991) revealed however, that although PEP produced a temporary increase in lung volume, this did not lead to an increase in the movement and clearance of mucus as evaluated by radio-aerosol technique (c.f. reduced lung volumes).
- Hofmeyr *et al.* (1986) performed a comparative trial between PEP/FET and ACBT. This study revealed no benefit in using the PEP mask. A greater quantity of sputum was cleared when using the ACBT.
- In the postoperative patient, the hourly use of PEP has been suggested to have 'prophylactic effects', reducing the risk of postoperative pulmonary complications (Ricksten *et al.* 1986, Richter Larsen *et al.* 1995).
- In stable CF (with scant sputum production), treatment with PEP increased functional residual capacity (c.f. reduced lung volumes). Air trapping decreased resulting in more evenly distributed peripheral ventilation (Groth *et al.* 1985). Compared to the Flutter device, PEP proved more effective in long-term maintenance of pulmonary function in a pediatric CF population (McIlwaine *et al.* 2001).
- For maximum efficacy, the patient aims to achieve between 10–20 cmH$_2$O pressure during mid-expiration (Falk & Anderson 1991).

- Twice daily treatment of 15 minutes duration is recommended for patients with stable lung disease (Falk & Anderson 1991).
- High pressure PEP (50–120 cmH$_2$O) is a modified form of the original modality, described by Oberwaldner *et al.* (1986) for the treatment of patients with cystic fibrosis. Individual optimum expiratory resistance should be determined with the use of spirometry prior to treatment.

Indications for use
- Removal of excess bronchial secretions.

Precautions
- PEP and high-pressure PEP may not be suitable adjuncts for use in patients at risk of air trapping (c.f. airflow limitation).

Contraindications
- PEP and high-pressure PEP should not be considered as a treatment modality in patients with frank hemoptysis.

Related topics

Impaired gaseous exchange (p. 44); Impaired tracheobronchial clearance (p. 48).

References and further reading

Falk M. and Anderson J.B. (1991) Positive expiratory pressure (PEP) mask. In: Pryor JA (ed) *Respiratory Care*. Churchill Livingstone, Edinburgh, pp. 51–63.

Falk M., Kelstrup M., Anderson J.B., Kinoshita T., Falk P., Stovring S., Gothgen I. (1984) Improving the ketchup bottle method with positive expiratory pressure, PEP, in cystic fibrosis. *Euro J Respir Dis* 65: 423–432.

Groth S., Stafanger G., Dirksen H., Andersen J.B., Falk M. and Kelstrup M. (1985) Positive expiratory pressure (PEP-mask) physiotherapy improves ventilation and reduces volume of trapped gas in cystic fibrosis. *Clin Respir Physiol* 21: 339–343.

Hofmeyr J.L., Webber B.A. and Hodson M.E. (1986) Evaluation of positive expiratory pressure as an adjunct to chest physiotherapy in the treatment of cystic fibrosis. *Thorax* 41: 951–954.

McIlwaine P.M., Wong L.T., Peacock D. and Davidson A.G. (2001) Long term comparative trial of PEP versus oscillatory PEP (Flutter) physiotherapy in the treatment of CF. *J Pediatr* 138(6): 845–850.

Oberwalder B., Evans J.C. and Zach M.S. (1986) Forced expirations against a variable resistance: a new chest physiotherapy method in cystic fibrosis. *Paediatric Pulmonol* 2: 358–367.

Richter Larsen K., Ingwersen U., Thode S. and Jakobsen S. (1995) Mask physiotherapy in patients after cardiac surgery: a controlled study. *Intens Care Med* 21(6): 467–468.

Ricksten S.E., Bengtsson A., Soderberg C., Thorden M. and Kvist H. (1986) Effects of periodic positive airway pressure by mask on post-operative pulmonary function. *Chest* 89: 774–781.

van der Schans C.P., van der Mark T.W., de Vries G. *et al.* (1991) Effect of positive pressure breathing in patients with cystic fibrosis. *Thorax* **46**: 252–256.

West J.B. (2000) *Respiratory Physiology – The Essentials*, 6th edition. Lippencott, Williams & Wilkins, Philadelphia.

THORACIC MOBILIZATIONS

Description

A passive accessory movement of any joint within the thorax, which the patient cannot actively perform. Passive oscillations are performed within or at the limit of the available range, in a manner that the rhythm and grade can be altered to achieve pain relief and restore function (Maitland 1986).

Key physiological principles

- Fibrous scar tissue may be laid down within the musculoskeletal system in response to an acute or chronic insult. If scar tissue is stressed at the correct time during its development the tissue formed has greater mobility and is less likely to restrict range of movement. Furthermore, when normal tissue extensibility is lost, fluid interchange is impaired and neurodynamics altered (Grieve 1981).
- The presence of articular mechanoreceptors and nociceptors are well documented. A function of the mechanoreceptor system is pain suppression, and consequently mobilizations may reduce pain by modulating nociceptive input (Lamb 1986).

Clinical relevance

Efficacy

- Early studies of thoracic mobilization techniques in patients with chronic respiratory disease suggest both subjective and objective improvements following treatment (Vibekk 1991).

Indications for use

- Clinically, musculoskeletal problems have been observed in patients secondary to cardiopulmonary dysfunction and vice versa. A thorough assessment is indicated in order to identify problems and formulate an appropriate treatment plan (c.f. assessment).
- The chest wall contributes to the loss in total respiratory system compliance in mechanically ventilated, acute respiratory failure patients (Katz *et al.* 1981). It is possible that thoracic mobilizations may be of benefit in addressing this problem (c.f. altered respiratory compliance).
- Characteristic changes in chest wall dimensions, muscle length and posture occur in the patient with chronic hyperinflation. Such individuals may experience pain and/or a reduction in vital capacity. Mobilization to thoracic joints may relieve associated pain (c.f. management of pain).
- Cardiac and thoracic surgery patients may experience painful limitation of thoracic mobility. Gentle mobilization techniques may be beneficial once postoperative bony union has occurred.

Application

- Commonly used techniques include postero-anterior central or unilateral vertebral pressures, transverse vertebral pressures, postero-anterior unilateral costovertebral pressures and sterno/costochondral joint mobilization. These techniques are intended to decrease pain and muscle spasm and improve mobility in joints and soft tissues.
- Treatment techniques may have to be modified if the patient cannot tolerate a starting position because of dyspnea or pain (c.f. positioning to relieve breathlessness).
- These techniques should not be used in isolation. Successful outcome depends upon maintenance of movement with muscle re-education and stretching, postural re-alignment, relaxation, self-mobilization techniques and advice (c.f. exercise training).
- Attention should also be paid to the cervical spine, scapulothoracic joints and glenohumeral joints.

Contraindications

- Contraindications to manual techniques include bony trauma, inflammation, infection or tumor, osteoporosis and neurological lesions.

Related topics

Chest wall deformity/disruption (p. 26); Infection and inflammation (p. 57); Pain and pain management (p. 58).

References and further reading

Grieve G.P. (1981) *Common Vertebral Joint Problems*. Churchill Livingstone, Edinburgh.

Katz J.A., Zinn S.E., Ozanne G.M. and Fairley H.B. (1981) Pulmonary, chest wall and lung-thorax elastances in acute respiratory failure. *Chest* **80**(3): 304–311.

Lamb D.W. (1986) A review of manual therapy for spinal pain: with reference to the lumbar spine. In: Grieve G.P. (ed) *Modern Manual Therapy of the Vertebral Column*. Churchill Livingstone, Edinburgh.

Maitland G.D. (1986) *Vertebral Manipulation*, 5th edition. Butterworth and Co., London.

Vibekk P. (1991) Chest mobilisation and respiratory function. In: Pryor J.A. (ed) *Respiratory Care*. Churchill Livingstone, Edinburgh.

TRACHEAL SUCTION

Description

Insertion of a catheter into the trachea to remove aspirate or excess bronchial secretions. Negative pressure (60–150 mmHg/8–20 kPa) is applied to the catheter to produce a suction effect. Access may be gained through a permanent tracheal stoma, tracheostomy tube, endotracheal tube, mini-tracheostomy, nasal or oral airway.

Key physiological principles

- In the absence of an intact cough reflex, tracheal suction will only remove secretions or aspirate located immediately around the end of the catheter.
- Suction can stimulate a cough reflex by direct mechanical stimulation of the larynx, carina, trachea or large bronchi (Widdicombe 1980).
- Effective coughing will mobilize secretions from more distal lung units, facilitating a greater yield with tracheal suction (Leith 1985).

Clinical relevance

Indications for use

- Tracheal suction is an invasive procedure, and therefore should only be undertaken when a clear indication has been identified through assessment.
- Indications for tracheal suction include an inability to cough effectively in the presence of retained secretions, or to assess endotracheal or tracheostomy tube patency.
- During physiotherapy treatment, tracheal suctioning is often used in combination with other techniques, e.g. manual hyperinflation, IPPB, exercise, ACBT, that assist in the mobilization of secretions (c.f. manual hyperinflation, IPPB, exercise training, ACBT).

Application

- Explaining the procedure of tracheal suctioning before starting treatment can reduce patient anxiety.
- Where nasal suction is indicated, insertion of a soft nasal airway prior to performing the procedure will maximize patient comfort.
- A sputum trap incorporated into the suction circuit allows the collection of a sterile specimen for microbiological assessment.
- Controversy exists regarding the instillation of normal saline prior to tracheal suction (Blackwood 1999). The only likely benefit of saline instillation is the stimulation of a cough reflex maximizing secretion mobilization and clearance (Raymond 1995) (c.f. impaired tracheobronchial clearance).
- Clinically, the use of 5 ml of normal saline has been shown to have no significant detrimental effect on hemodynamics, respiratory mechanics or gas exchange (Gray *et al.* 1990).

- The size of the suction catheter selected should be less than half the diameter of the airway or endotracheal/tracheostomy tube (Rosen & Hillard 1962).
- Multi-eyed suction catheters are most effective at removing secretions and cause least mechanical trauma (Jung & Gottlieb 1976).
- Careful insertion of the catheter is imperative as the majority of mucosal damage may occur during this stage (Kleiber *et al.* 1988). On insertion, the catheter should be introduced either until a resistance is felt or a cough reflex has been elicited. Before suction is applied, the catheter should be withdrawn 1 cm.
- Closed-circuit suction systems consisting of a catheter enclosed in a sterile sheath are commercially available (Quirke 1997). This system avoids disconnection ·from the ventilator; minimizing interruption of ventilation, oxygenation and PEEP, which may reduce hypoxia induced arrhythmias (c.f. mechanical ventilation). Indications for use; high-risk infection, copious secretions, high levels of PEEP or supplemental oxygen.

Precautions
- Hypoxemia induced during suction can be attributed to apnea, or the removal of oxygen from the airway along with secretions. Pre-oxygenating the patient before suction begins and limiting the duration of the suction procedure can minimize hypoxemia.
- Cardiac arrhythmias are more common in the presence of hypoxia.
- In most normal adult subjects, tracheal stimulation produces increased sympathetic nervous system activity. However, in some instances tracheal stimulation during suction may cause a vasovagal reflex producing cardiac arrhythmias and hypotension (Young 1984). This response is commonly seen in patients following spinal cord injury above the level of T_1, as sympathetic dominance is lost (Frankel *et al.* 1975).
- During tracheal suction the removal of air from the lungs may produce closure of small airways. This may be particularly problematic in patients with a high closing capacity (c.f. reduced lung volumes). This problem can be minimized by adequate lung inflation after suctioning (Mansell *et al.* 1972) (c.f. manual hyperinflation, IPPB, ACBT).
- Tracheal suction can introduce infection to the patient. There is also a potential risk of infection to the therapist. Local infection control policies should be adhered to.
- Poor technique and a badly designed or selected suction catheter can induce mucosal trauma.
- There is an associated risk of vomiting with oral suction.

Contraindications
- Absolute contraindications to tracheal suctioning are unexplained hemoptysis, severe coagulopathies, severe bronchospasm, laryngeal stridor or a compromised cardiovascular system.
- Nasal or oral suction should not be performed in a patient with a known basal skull fracture, or CSF leakage via the ear.

- Tracheal suctioning has been shown to increase ICP (Young 1984), but most elevations are transient and return to baseline values within minutes. However, patients with cerebral irritation may not conform to this response. Consequently, an absolute indication for suctioning must be identified before proceeding.

Related topics

Impaired tracheobronchial clearance (p. 48); Manual hyperinflation (p. 102); Tracheostomy management (p. 148).

References and further reading

Blackwood B. (1999) Normal saline instillation with endotracheal suctioning: primum non nocere (first do no harm). *J Adv Nurs* **29**: 928–934.

Frankell H.L., Mathias C.J. and Spalding J.M. (1975) Mechanisms of reflex cardiac arrest in tetraplegic patients. *Lancet* **2**: 1183–1185.

Gray J.E., MacIntyre N.R. and Kronenberger W.G. (1990) The effects of bolus normal saline instillation in conjunction with endotracheal suctioning. *Respiratory Care* **35**: 785–790.

Jung R.C. and Gottlieb L.S. (1976) Comparison of tracheo-bronchial suction catheters in humans. *Chest* **69**: 170–181.

Kleiber C., Krutzfield N. and Rose E.F. (1988) Acute histologic changes in the tracheo-bronchial tree associated with different suction catheter insertion techniques. *Heart Lung* **17**: 10–14.

Leith D.E. (1985) The development of cough. *Am Rev Respir Dis* **131**: S39–42.

Mansell A., Bryan C. and Levison H. (1972) Airway closure in children. *J Appl Physiol* **33**: 711–714.

Quirke S. (1997) Closed circuit suction systems. *Care Critic Ill* **13** (suppl): 6.

Raymond S.J. (1995) Normal saline instillation before suctioning; helpful or harmful? *Am J Crit Care* **4**: 267–271.

Rosen M. and Hillard E.K. (1962) The effects of negative pressure during tracheal suction. *Anesth Analg (Cleave)* **41**: 50–57.

Widdicombe J.G. (1980) Mechanism of cough and its regulation. *Euro J Respir Dis* **61** (Suppl 110): 11–15.

Young C.S. (1984) A review of the adverse effects of airway suction. *Physiotherapy* **70**: 104–106.

TRACHEOSTOMY MANAGEMENT

Description

The formation of a stoma in the anterior wall of the trachea. The procedure may be surgical, percutaneous or via a cricothyroidotomy (for mini-tracheostomy insertion).

Key physiological principles

- A formal tracheostomy reduces upper airway anatomical dead space, which decreases the work of breathing and increases alveolar ventilation.

Types of tracheostomy tube

Cuffed tubes	For patients requiring positive pressure ventilatory support, or at risk of aspiration. Cuff pressure should be <25 mmHg to minimize pressure trauma. NB Cuff may be deflated for the purposes of tracheostomy weaning.
Uncuffed tubes	Commonly used for children (<10 years) as air leaks are minimal, or long-term stomas.
Tubes with an inner cannulae (double lumen)	The inner tube may be removed for cleaning, thereby reducing the risk of tube occlusion with encrusted secretions. Single lumen tubes should be changed after 10 days, double lumen tubes within 1 month.
Fenestrated double lumen tube	An aperture in the upper aspect of the tracheostomy tube allows passage of air via the mouth, nose and vocal cords, facilitating the weaning process. May be utilized as a nonfenestrated tube by using a nonfenestrated inner tube if necessary.

Clinical relevance

Indications for use

- Provides airway access for long-term ventilation (c.f. mechanical ventilation, NIPPV).
- Allows a controlled mechanical ventilation weaning program to be performed in a conscious patient.
- Relief of upper airway obstruction/stricture.
- Prevention of aspiration with persistent swallowing impairment.
- Removal of excessive sputum retention. NB A mini-tracheostomy is usually performed for the purposes of secretion removal only (c.f. impaired tracheobronchial clearance).
- Following oral, facial or neck injuries.

Complications

- hemorrhage;
- misplacement, blockage or occlusion;
- pneumothorax;
- bronchospasm;
- unplanned extubation;
- infection;
- tracheal (± esophageal) damage.

Maintenance

- Humidification is essential as the upper airway is bypassed (c.f. humidification).
- The need for suction must be assessed on an individual patient basis (c.f. suction). Ideally, suction should not be attempted with a fenestrated inner tube *in situ*, unless it is multifenestrated (with small apertures) and therefore will not allow the suction catheter to pass through and damage the tracheal wall.
- Tube encrustation may be minimized by use of double lumen tubes. The inner cannulae should be checked frequently and rinsed (sterile water or 0.9% saline) or replaced. Brushes should not be used as they may damage the surface of the inner tube, promoting bacterial colonization.
- Occlusion of the tracheostomy tube is a life-threatening situation. Causes include encrusted secretions, tube misplacement, cuff herniation, or iatrogenic (e.g. capping off a non-fenestrated tracheostomy with the cuff inflated).
- Signs of tube occlusion include respiratory distress, tachycardia, anxiety, desaturation, absence/reduction of flow via tracheostomy tube on exhalation, etc.
- In the event of a tube occlusion help must be sought immediately. Position the patient with their head in a mid-line position, clear secretions as able, replace the inner tube if possible, deflate the cuff and administer oxygen via a face mask. If the tube is completely occluded it will require removal and replacement with a new tracheostomy tube or endotracheal tube. If tube insertion fails or is not possible, mask-stoma or face-mask ventilation (with the stoma occluded) will be required.

Precautions

- Emergency equipment must be kept at the patient's bedside including spare tracheostomy tube (same size plus one smaller), 10 ml syringe, tracheal dilators, suction equipment/unit, forceps, a rebreathing circuit and Ambu Bag.
- Hygiene is essential; all attending personnel should apply universal precautions prior to any intervention.

Tracheostomy and speech

- The tracheostomized patient should be offered the appropriate means to communicate, e.g. picture boards, pen and paper, electronic devices.
- Vocalization may be possible using one-way speaking valves or intermittent finger occlusion with the cuff deflated. Fenestrated tubes also allow for vocalization, ideally with the cuff deflated to prevent excessive work of breathing.

- If there is evidence or likelihood of aspiration a referral to the speech and language therapist (SALT) should be made. A comprehensive swallow assessment can only be made when the tracheostomy tube cuff is deflated.
- During tests for cuff deflation, vocalization and swallowing the patient's condition, including oxygen saturation, must be closely monitored.

Weaning and decannulation

- For successful weaning the patient must be optimized both medically and psychologically.
- Initially, the patient may tolerate <5 min with the cuff deflated, but this should gradually be increased.
- When deflating the tracheostomy tube cuff, it is advisable to simultaneously suction in the oropharynx to prevent aspiration of secretions, which may have collected above the cuff (c.f. suction).
- Once the patient can tolerate several hours of cuff deflation, the process may be repeated with a decannulation cap occluding the tracheostomy opening.
- The decision to change or decannulate must be made by a competent practitioner and/or attending medical staff. The procedure should only be undertaken by a suitably trained individual with advanced airway management skills.

Related topics

Impaired tracheobronchial clearance (p. 48); Respiratory failure (p. 63); Respiratory muscle dysfunction (p. 66).

References and further reading

St. George's Healthcare NHS Trust (2000) *Guidelines for the Care of Patients with Tracheostomy Tubes.* Sims Portex Ltd., Hythe, Kent.

Section 4

CASE STUDIES AND SELF-ASSESSMENT

CASE STUDY 1

A 35-year-old known asthmatic man has just been admitted to the medical ward with a 2-day history of fever, cough productive of sputum and left-sided chest pain.

> PMH: asthmatic;
>
> DH: salbutamol and beclothemasone via metered dose inhalers;
>
> SH: computer programmer lives with wife;
>
> O/E:
>
> - Temperature 39°C;
> - Tachypneic RR 30, SOBAR talking in clipped sentences, shallow breaths;
> - Auscultation: reduced breath sounds bi-basally, inspiratory crackles left lower lobe, faint monophonic expiratory wheeze left lower lobe;
> - CXR: Patchy white shadowing LL zone;
> - ABGs: (F_iO_2 0.4) pH 7.48, PCO_2 4.4, PO_2 10.5, HCO_3^- 25 BE −1.

What pathophysiology can be identified?

What are the underlying causal factors?

Physiotherapy treatment

CASE STUDY 1 SOLUTION

What pathophysiology can be identified?

- Acid–base disturbance: respiratory alkalosis with hypoxemia.
- Airflow limitation: expiratory wheeze.
- Impaired gas exchange: hypoxemia.
- Probable infection: pyrexia, productive of sputum, CXR shadowing.
- Impaired tracheobronchial clearance: retained secretions.
- Pain: pleuritic chest pain.
- Reduced lung volume: Reduced basal BS on auscultation ?bi-basal atelectasis on CXR, altered respiratory pattern.

What are the underlying causal factors?

- Acid–base disturbance: hypoxemia secondary to pulmonary infiltrate, probable infection, producing V/Q mismatch. RR raised to compensate for hypoxemia producing a fall in CO_2. Renal compensation has not occurred.
- Airflow limitation: local airway inflammation producing narrowing or sputum-related obstruction.
- Impaired gas exchange: large pulmonary infiltrate producing an area of low V/Q 'wasted perfusion'. Patient is unable to compensate for this by increasing RR. Collapse of lung units distal to site of infection will contribute to ongoing hypoxemia.
- Infection: probable respiratory infection, microorganism as yet unknown.
- Pain: pleuritis secondary to probable infection.
- Reduced lung volume: Reduced V_T secondary to pain. Atelectasis of lung units distal to site of infection.

Physiotherapy treatment

- Acid–base disturbance: Positioning to relieve SOB, breathing control to normalize RR. Oxygen therapy (prescribed by doctor) optimize delivery with correct device, humidification.
- Airflow limitation: bronchodilator therapy, nebulized rather than MDI (prescribed by doctor).
- Impaired gaseous exchange: position patient to maximize V/Q.
- Probable infection: if possible send sputum specimen for cytology.
- Impaired tracheobronchial clearance: positioning to relieve SOB, mucociliary clearance techniques: ACBT +/– manual techniques, GAP.
- Pain: TNS, analgesia (prescribed by doctor).
- Reduced lung volume: adjunct to increase V_T and assist expectoration, e.g. IPPB, adjunct to increase FRC and assist re-expansion of atelectasis, e.g. CPAP. NB caution should be exercised in acute stage to reduce risk of further air trapping. Advise patient on positioning to improve lung volumes and promote early mobilization.

CASE STUDY 2

A 65-year-old man is 2 days post-operative following surgery for four coronary artery by-pass grafts. He was extubated in recovery and returned to the high-dependency unit. Over the past 6 hours his RR and O_2 requirements have increased. He is sweating and complaining of sternal chest pain. BP 110/55, F_iO_2 0.5.

PMH: ischaemic heart disease with angina;
MI 18/12 ago.

SH: 20/day for 30 years. Stopped 5 years ago;
exercise tolerance 200 yards on flat;
sleeps with 3 pillows.

O/E:

- Obese;
- Low-grade pyrexia 37.8°C;
- tachypneic RR 35;
- palpation: reduced chest expansion L>R. Dull to percussion L base, with decreased vocal resonance/tactile vocal fremitus;
- auscultation: reduced breath sounds bi-basally L>R, scattered basal crackles;
- CXR: bi-basal plate atelectasis with moderate L-sided pleural effusion;
- ABGs: (F_iO_2 0.5) pH 7.49, PCO_2 4.5, PO_2 9.8, HCO_3^- 22 BE –4.

What pathophysiology can be identified?

What are the underlying causal factors?

Physiotherapy treatment

CASE STUDY 2 SOLUTION

What pathophysiology can be identified?

- Acid–base disturbance: respiratory alkalosis with hypoxemia.
- Altered respiratory compliance: atelectasis, sternal chest pain.
- Chest wall dysfunction: sternal split.
- Impaired gaseous exchange: hypoxemia, increased F_iO_2 requirements.
- Pain: sternal chest pain.
- Reduced lung volume: plate atelectasis on CXR, reduced BS on auscultation, altered respiratory pattern.
- Deconditioning: poor exercise tolerance.

What are the underlying causal factors?

- Acid–base disturbance: hypoxemia secondary to bi-basal atelectasis producing V/Q mismatch. RR raised to compensate for hypoxemia producing a fall in CO_2. Renal compensation has occurred.
- Altered respiratory compliance: sternal split, altered thoracic mobility, moderate L-sided pleural effusion, atelectasis, effects of GA, pain, ?some degree of heart failure, obesity.
- Chest wall dysfunction: sternal split.
- Impaired gaseous exchange: bi-basal atelectasis producing an area of low V/Q 'wasted perfusion'. Patient is unable to fully compensate for this by increasing RR.
- Pain: sternal split, ?peri-operative MI.
- Reduced lung volume: reduced FRC secondary to GA and obesity, reduced V_T secondary to pain.
- Deconditioning: known ischemic heart disease, recent MI.

Physiotherapy treatment

- Acid–base disturbance: oxygen therapy (prescribed by doctor), optimize delivery with correct device, humidification, positioning to relieve SOB and optimize diaphragmatic function.
- Altered respiratory compliance: stabilize sternum with 'cough-lock' or draw sheet, ?discuss drainage of effusion with medical team, ?some pulmonary edema discuss diuretic therapy with medical team, position patient to release abdomen forwards and optimize diaphragmatic function, pain relief (see below), reversal of atelectasis (see below), when clinically stable mobilize thoracic joints as appropriate.
- Chest wall dysfunction: stabilize sternum with 'cough-lock' or draw sheet.
- Impaired gaseous exchange: Position to optimize V/Q ratio.
- Pain: discuss with medical team to eliminate peri-operative MI, analgesia prescribed by doctor.
- Reduced lung volume: adjunct to increase V_T and assist expectoration of possible retained secretions, e.g. IPPB, adjunct to increase FRC and assist re-expansion of atelectasis, e.g. CPAP. Positioning to improve lung volumes as

tolerated. NB note this patient's borderline hypotension before applying positive pressure device, discuss need for pharmacological intervention with medical team.

- Deconditioning: start early mobilization program when appropriate. On-going cardiac rehabilitation program on discharge.

CASE STUDY 3

A 48-year-old woman admitted to the ITU 3/52 ago. She developed ARDS secondary to biliary sepsis following cholecystectomy. She is mechanically ventilated via a tracheostomy using a lung protective strategy. She has a history of bilateral pneumothoraces and has multiple chest drains *in situ*, none of which are presently bubbling. In the last 24 hours gas exchange has deteriorated requiring an increased F_iO_2. In addition she has required the introduction of inotropic support. She has a fever and is now productive of sputum, and has developed a new pulmonary infiltrate on CXR. The patient's WCC is elevated.

> DH: noradrenaline (0.15 mg per kg), heparin (2500 IU s.c.) ranitidine.
>
> O/E:
>
> - temperature 38.5°C;
> - BP 105/58, HR 105;
> - CVP 12, PAP 50/25, PCOP 15;
> - FiO_2 0.7;
> - ABGs: pH 7.2, PCO_2 9, PO_2 9.2, HCO_3^- 31, BE +5;
> - ventilation: Pressure-controlled ventilation 25, PEEP 10, I:E ratio 1:1, RR 18, V_T 350 ml;
> - CXR: diffuse bilateral interstitial shadowing, consolidation R lower zone.

What pathophysiology can be identified?

What are the underlying causal factors?

Physiotherapy treatment

CASE STUDY 3 SOLUTION

What pathophysiology can be identified?

- Acid–base disturbance: respiratory acidosis with hypoxemia.
- Altered respiratory compliance: ARDS, pneumothorax, consolidation.
- Deconditioning: long-term mechanical ventilation.
- Disorders of pulmonary circulation: interstitial fluid/edema.
- Impaired gaseous exchange: hypoxemia, increasing F_iO_2 requirement.
- Impaired tracheobronchial clearance: productive of sputum, intubated.
- Infection: pyrexia, sputum production, increasing WCC.
- Sepsis/SIRS: previous surgery.
- Reduced lung volume: ARDS, long-term mechanical ventilation supine position.

What are the underlying causal factors?

- Acid–base disturbance: Respiratory alkalosis secondary to ventilator strategy. Hypoxemia secondary to infective pulmonary infiltrate (consolidation), producing V/Q mismatch. Due to the use of a 'protective lung' ventilator strategy, V_T cannot be raised to compensate for hypoxemia as permissive hypercapnia is being employed. Renal compensation has occurred.
- Altered respiratory compliance: In the resolution phase of ARDS abnormal collagen is laid down producing fibrosis and reduced compliance. The presence of a pneumothorax represents disruption of the lung surface and a subsequent alteration in pleural pressure, reducing lung compliance. Consolidation is an expanded airless area, which no longer retains elastic properties altering compliance.
- Deconditioning: In as little as 24 h, immobility and recumbency has an influence on many body systems. Long-term ventilation may result in muscle atrophy, tendon shortening, a reduced range of joint motion, demineralization of bones and generalized deconditioning.
- Impaired gaseous exchange: Infective consolidation R lower zone producing an area of low V/Q 'wasted perfusion'. Patient is unable to compensate for this by increasing V_T. Collapse of lung units distal to site of infection will contribute to ongoing hypoxemia.
- Impaired tracheobronchial clearance: patient sedated and intubated for 3 weeks leading to suppressed cough reflex.
- Infection: Nosocomial infection organism as yet unknown.
- Sepsis/SIRS: Sepsis developed following cholecystectomy.
- Reduced lung volume: Patient receiving 'protective lung' ventilator strategy, therefore, V_T is reduced. Atelectasis may occur in lung units distal to site of infection/consolidation.

Physiotherapy treatment

- Altered respiratory compliance: MHI, Thoracic mobilization.
- Deconditioning: Accurate positioning and movement of all limbs and available joints. An early progressive mobilization program when appropriate.

- Impaired gaseous exchange: a regular change of position to maximize V/Q ratio as tolerated by the patient. Consider prone positioning.
- Impaired tracheobronchial clearance: Modified GAP, MHI +/– saline installation suction, as tolerated. NB Note hypotension, discuss with medical team the need for a bolus of inotropic support. Note high F_iO_2 requirement and consider recovery strategy should patient desaturate. Note if the patient is 'PEEP dependent', the use of closed-circuit suction is advocated.
- Infection: if possible send sputum specimen for cytology.
- Reduced lung volume: MHI to increase V_T and mobilize secretions, reduce airway resistance and recruit lung units via channels of collateral ventilation. A subsequent increase in FRC may be noted. The use of a 'PEEP valve' may help preserve PEEP during MHI.
- Tracheostomy management: to ensure tube patency and effective removal of secretions. Check efficacy of humidification device. The introduction of a speaking tube when appropriate.

CASE STUDY 4

A 55-year-old woman with a kyphoscoliosis presents with a 4/52 history of increased SOBOE, general lethargy, headaches and swelling of the lower limbs. Prior to this admission she considered herself to be fit and well. However, for the past few years she complains of feeling 'a little chesty', for which her GP has prescribed inhalers.

DH: salbutamol MDI, ipratropium bromide MDI, frusemide.

SH: Lives alone, 1st floor flat, previously independent.
Decreasing exercise tolerance over the past year.

O/E:

- Apyrexial;
- RR 28;
- asymmetric chest movement consistent with kyphoscoliosis;
- reduced breath sounds R base consistent with kyphoscoliosis;
- ABGs: (F_iO_2 0.28) pH 7.38, pCO_2 8.0, pO_2 8.5, HCO_3^- 34, BE +8;
- CXR: consistent with kyphoscoliosis, no additional infiltrates.

What pathophysiology can be identified?

What are the underlying causal factors?

Physiotherapy treatment

CASE STUDY 4 SOLUTION

What pathophysiology can be identified?
- Chest wall disruption/deformity: kyphoscoliosis.
- Respiratory failure: hypercapnia and hypoxia.
- Heart failure: 'chesty', swelling of lower limbs.
- Deconditioning: reduced exercise tolerance.

What are the underlying causal factors?
- Chest wall disruption/deformity: congenital kyphoscoliosis.
- Respiratory failure: type II or ventilatory failure secondary to restrictive lung disease associated with kyphoscoliosis.
- Heart failure: cor pulmonale.
- Deconditioning: associated with restrictive lung disease and cor pulmonale.

Physiotherapy treatment
- Chest wall disruption/deformity: Thoracic mobilizations may help increase thoracic mobility and chest wall compliance.
- Respiratory failure: Position to relieve breathlessness. Application of NIPPV titrated to relieve hypercapnia with sufficient O_2 entrained to reverse hypoxemia. Adequate humidification should be included in the circuit. NB A sleep study may be necessary for accurate titration, to prevent the development of nocturnal hypercapnia.
- Heart failure: Symptomatic relief may be gained from beneficial effects of NIPPV. Discuss with medical team to increase diuretic dose.
- Deconditioning: Positioning to increase lung volumes. Implement an early mobilization program starting on NIPPV and progressing to self-ventilating with O_2 when appropriate. When clinically stable commence pulmonary rehabilitation program.

INDEX